NATUROPATHY

NATUROPATHY

For Perfect Health

Editor

S.D. Dwivedi

PUBLICATIONS

KALPAZ PUBLICATIONS

DELHI-110052

NATUROPATHY: For Perfect Health

(Health)

RS. 290/-

ISBN : 81-7835-075-0

Published in 2002 in India by

Kalpaz Publications
C-30, Satyawati Nagar
Delhi-110052

E-mail: kalpaz@hotmail.com

Laser Typesetting : A.S. Printers, Delhi

Printed at : Mehra Offset Press, Delhi

CONTENTS

PREFACE

Today we are very well aware of the numerous side-effects of the modern drugs, environmental pollution chemical fertilizers, food, modern life style, stressful life, hence, we are gradually losing faith in conventional therapeutic systems. Nature itself is the healer and we should keep it in our minds that it has given us such a system which can fight with diseases in an efficient manner. The gifts of nature like air, water, sunlight, etc., are free so why should not we utilise them?

Nature cure is not new to India, it has been in use since ages as an effective science, and in modern times millions of people in India and many other countries are being benefited by it.

Naturopathy does not harm the patient in any way. After trying various methods described in this book, you will find that they are quite simple and extremely effective. However, before applying any method read instructions carefully, because it is essential to understand the correct method to ensure better results. I hope that the readers will derive tremendous benefit from this book and deal with diseases in a natural way. Their houses without spending lot of money and time in lostly medicines and other medical charges like doctor's fees, nursing home charges etc.

S.D. Dwivedi

Some Suggestions

* Nothing except water should be consumed when you are fasting. The intake of water should be two to two and a half litres.
* In the evening of the first day of the fast and the morning after, an enema of hot water should be taken.
* A day's, fasting should be followed by a food intake 25 per cent less than one normally consumes.
* A two day's, fast should be followed by consumption of fruits only next day. Usual diet should follow next day—after fruit diet for a day.
* A three day's, fast should be followed the next day by fruit juices and soup of vegetables, the soup must be without addition of any thickening agents or condiments. On the fifth day eat fruits only and on the sixth breakfast on fruits, lunch on bread and boiled vegetables and repeat a fruit diet for dinner. Afterwards you may resume your normal intake of food.

CHAPTER 1

Fasting for Cleanse Process

Fasting is one of the best tools that Naturopathy uses in the battle against all kind of diseases. The presence of germs in the body is only a symptom of a disease, not its cause.

If there is accumulation of acid and toxic substances in the body, only then the diseases may launch attack on it. The efforts of the body to get rid of these harmful substances are what we deem to be the symptoms of diseases. When the poisons accumulate beyond the normal limits in the body, the body makes strenuous and violent efforts to eliminate them. It is these constructive efforts that are mistakenly regarded as acute diseases. The body concentrates all its energies on the process of healing. In these circumstances, the body does not need food. This results in loss of appetite, and there is a foul taste in the mouth. If something is consumed at such a time, the energy of the body gets diverted to the process of digestion. Consequently, the elimination of poisons is stalled, and the disease intensifies.

Sometimes fasting becomes a little difficult. A patient suffering from some ailment may declare unequivocally that he is not hungry, and there is a bitter taste in his mouth. But family members, and well-wishers keep on insisting for something like tea, coffee, milk, fruit juice, porridge, etc. They keep urging the patient, and do not rest till he takes something. The patient is thus compelled to eat, despite his complete disinclination. The food remains undigested, adds to the burden on the system, and illness is prolonged. In fact, man is the only creature that continues to eat even when indisposed, and even when he has no appetite. You must have noticed that no other animal eats if it is sick.

Most of the people believe that if they forego even one meal in a day, they will become undernourished and die prematurely. This notion is ridiculous. Food taken in illness nourishes the illness, not the sufferer, hence it is better to avoid food if one has no desire.

The persons who are accustomed to make do occasionally with only one meal a day would find fasting for one or two days quite easy. Similarly, those who are accustomed to fasting for one or two days from time to time will not be deterred or feel inconvenience in four or five day's fast, or even more longer ones.

This is very difficult to estimate beforehand the period of fasting required in cases of long-standing and pernicious disorders. It is, therefore, advisable that fasting for extended periods be supervised by an expert. For really long periods of fasting, it is necessary to check the blood and urine of the patient frequently. If ketones are found to be present in the urine or the amount of urea in the blood is found to exceed 45 mg per cent, then the fast should be discontinued at once.

The fasts should be terminated in the proper manner, this is more important than the fast itself. The digestive organs have become relaxed during the fast. If discretion is not exercised in the quality and quantity of food after a fast, the inevitable result is that the digestive system is unable to cope with the sudden increase in the intake of food, and the digestive process remains incomplete, leading to the generation of toxic substances. This may cause fresh invasion of disease.

Fever, cold, cough, flu and most other similar diseases are cured by only two to three days' fasting. Where long-standing or chronic diseases are concerned, fasting should be planned with some care and foresight, as longer periods of fasting are necessary. In such cases, one must take light uncooked or liquid diet for three to four days prior to the commencement of the fasting period. This initiates the process of the purification of the blood. Moreover, vitamins and minerals obtained from the raw foods are stored in the body, which prove to be quite useful later during the period of fasting.

If one does not follow this rule strictly, then the fast itself may prove futile, and may even cause harm. Fasting becomes necessary in the first place only because of failure to maintain regularity, propriety and proportion in food habits. If the same irregularity impropriety and thoughtlessness are to be indulged in after a fast as before it, the body can once again become a godown of poisons, and therefore subject to the consequent complications.

Even if a healthy person regularly undertakes fasting for one day in every ten or twelve days it purifies the body, and thus can keep away the diseases.

CHAPTER 2

Diet for Better Health

The diet in naturopathy is of great importance, because its most of the treatment consists of cleansing the system through diet. The approach of allopaths towards diet is rather casual. They advise diet that contains the requisite proportions of proteins, carbohydrates, fats, vitamins and minerals. But most of the doctors are not care much about the diet of their patients. If a patient asks for advice in this regard, he is likely to be told that there are no specific restrictions, he can have a balanced diet.

Eating should be necessary function as breathing, but it should not be adopted by people as means of gratifying their desire for the nice things of life. In Ayurveda, all foods are classified into categories like phlegm-promoting or phlegm-destroying, bile-promoting or bile-destroying and gas-promoting or gas-destroying. To some extent, foods are also differentiated as heavy or light foods. Ayurveda had its origin thousands of years ago, when methods and equipment had not yet been developed for the analysis of foods. Ayurveda had no means of ascertaining what biochemical reactions took place in the body due to the ingestion of various foods. Its emphasis on the liberal consumption of pure ghee, oil, crystal sugar and spiced health-foods is incorrect and outdated. There also seems to be an excessive bias in favour of cooked foods.

Proper diet is very important in naturopathic treatment. In this system, a detailed study has been made of the merits and demerits of each food and drink. Proper diet can be a veritable elixir of life, turning one into lush of health. Improper diet, on the other hand, can act as a poison, destroying health and life as well.

Food is required for supplying all essential nutrients to the body and maintain the acid-alkali balance in the blood.

The main ingredients of foods essential for the nutrition of the body are proteins, carbohydrates, fats, minerals and vitamins.

Proteins

Proteins are essential for the maintenance, growth and regeneration of the body. The main sources of proteins are milk, eggs, meat, pulses, etc. All proteins are made up of amino acids and different proteins contain different proportions of different amino acids.

There are in all twenty-three amino acids in food proteins. Out of these, there are ten that the human body cannot synthesize: histidine, isoleucine, leucine, arginine, valine, methionine, phenylalanine, threonine, tryptophane and lysine. These are essential amino acids. The body must be supplied with the requisite amounts of these amino acids through food. The rest of the amino acids can be synthesized by the body from these. The functions of each of the amino acid in the body is given in the following table along with their sources.

S. No.	Amino Acid	Body part where it is required	Sources
1.	Cystine	Erythrocytes, breasts, vitality, hair	Alfalfa, apples, carrots, beetroots, cabbages, cauliflower, onions, garlic, pineapples, raspberries, raisins.
2.	Arginine	Cartilage cells, reproductive organs, prevention of senility, muscles	Alfalfa, green leafy vegetables, carrots, beetroots cucumber, celery, lettuce, potatoes, radishes.
3.	Aspartic acid	Bones, blood vessels, teeth, lungs, heart	Apples, almonds, celery, cucumber, carrots, mint, radishes, tomatoes, turnips, lemons, grapefruit, plums, pineapples, melons.
4.	Alanine	Adrenal glands, skin	Almonds, alfalfa, carrots, celery, lettuce, cucumber, green pepper, spinach, apples, plums, guavas, grapes, oranges, strawberries, turnips.
5.	Glutamic acid	Secretion of digestive juices, prevention of anaemia, pancreas	Carrots, cabbages, celery, beetroots, mint, lettuce, spinach, papaya, turnips
6.	Lodogorgoic acid	Various glands	Celery, spinach, carrots, tomatoes, lettuce, pineapples.
7.	Histidine	Haemoglobin, semen, liver	Carrots, beetroots, radishes, celery, cucumber, garlic, onions, turnips, alfalfa, spinach, pineapples, pomegranates, papaya, apple.

(Contd.)

8.	Hydroxygluta-mic acid	Secretion of digestive juices	Mint, lettuce, spinach, carrots, tomatoes, grapes, plums, raspberries.
9.	Hydroxy proline	Gall bladder, erythrocytes, liver	Beetroots, lettuce, carrots, turnips, cucumber, plums, cherries, figs, radishes, grapes, olives, almonds, coconuts, pineapples.
10.	Glycine	Muscles, secretion of sex hormones, cartilage cells	Carrots, celery, mint, spinach, alfalfa, garlic, potatoes, figs, oranges, raspberries, pomegranates, melons, almonds, turnips.
11.	Isoleucine	Spleen, pituitary gland, haemoglobin, regulation of metabolism, thymus	Coconuts, almonds, apricots, pistachios, walnuts, papaya, olives.
12.	Leucine	Counterbalancing isoleucine	Coconut, papaya, olives, almonds, apricots, pista-chios, walnuts.
13.	Norleucine	Counterbalan-cing leucine	
14.	Methionine	Spleen, pancreas, haemoglobin	Cauliflower, cabbages, garlic, apples, pineapples.
15.	Lysine	Fat metabolism, various processes in the body, prevention of senility, liver, gall bladder	Beetroots, cucumber, carrots, celery, mint, spinach, turnips, pears, alfalfa, germinated soyabeans, papaya, apples, plums, grapes.

(Contd.)

16.	Phenylalanine	Elimination of foreign substa-nces, urinary bladder, kidneys	Beetroots, spinach, carrots, mint, tomatoes, apples, pineapples.
17.	Proline	White blood corpuscles (leucocytes)	Beetroots, lettuce, carrots turnips, cucumber, cherries, grapes, olives, oranges, pineapples, coconuts, almonds, figs.
18.	Valine	Ovaries, breasts	Carrots, sweet gourd, celery, mint, beetroots, tomatoes, turnips, apples, pomegranates, almonds.
19.	Threonine	To make good the deficiency of some other amino acids	Alfalfa, green leafy vege-tables, papaya, carrots.
20.	Thyroxine	Thyroid, pituitary glands, adrenal glands, regulation of metabolism	Celery, lettuce, spinach, carrots, turnips, tomat-oes, pineapples.
21.	Tryptophane	Regeneration of cells, secretion of digestive juices, eyes	Beetroots, celery, carrots, spinach, alfalfa, turnips.
22.	Tyrosine	Hair, adrenal, pituitary and thyroid glands, erythrocytes, leucocytes	Beetroots, alfalfa, carrots, cucumber, lettuce, mint, spinach, green pepper, plums, strawbe-rries, cherries, apples, melons, almonds, figs.
23.	Serine	Mucous membranes, bronchi, lungs	Radishes, onions, carrots, garlic, beetroots, celery, cucumber, mint, spinach, cabbage, alfalfa,papaya, apples, pineapples.

This is common belief that animal proteins are superior and indeed complete food proteins, or best proteins, whereas vegetable proteins are inferior, incomplete and 'second class' proteins. This belief is based on the fact that meat contains all the essential amino acids, but any one specific vegetable food does not contain all of them. Many nutritionists, therefore, advise people to take meat in one form or the other. They insist on vegetarians taking plenty of milk, so that they can get sufficient amounts of superior proteins and the body can remain healthy.

However, this emphasis on animal proteins, whether in the form of meat or milk, is incorrect. By combining vegetable proteins in proper proportions, we can get all the essential amino acids in the requisite amounts. One food may lack valine, but may contain enough of lysine. Another one may lack lysine, but may supply all the valine required. Thus, by a judicious blending of foodstuffs, the deficiency of any amino acid can be compensated for. For instance, if wheaten foods are combined with vegetables, the combination yields proteins of the best quality. Hence,this belief that a vegetarian is likely to suffer from the deficiency of one or more essential amino acids has no ground. That superior proteins are available in animal food is also a fact, but it must be remembered that there are numerous drawbacks attached to the use of such foods, because they lead to many other complications.

There are excessive amounts of proteins in a non-vegetarian diet. An excess of proteins is doubtlessly the chief factor in the invasion of many diseases. The famous dietician, an expert, states that

> "ingestion of excessive amounts of proteins results in the formation of uric acid, which is harmful to health Many of the diseases troubling mankind have their roots in the excessive intake of proteins."

Another expert says that when too much of protein enters the blood stream, it gets converted into nitric acid sulphuric acid and phosphoric acid. The body is forced to use up large amounts of alkali minerals to neutralize these acids. This results in a deficiency of minerals in the bones, hair and nails. The acids mentioned above cause so much damage to the liver and the kidneys that in some cases it may even prove deadly. He concluded that diseases are less prevalent in countries where the consumption of proteinous foods is low. He forcefully asserted that no adult wishing to live a long and healthy life should take more than twenty grammes of proteins per day.

Another expert attributes the rise in the proportion of deaths due to Bright's disease in America and other developed countries solely to excessive consumption of meat.

A team of experts thoroughly investigated the effect of protein-rich foods on the kidneys. In one experiment they began to feed each of five healthy men half a kilogramme of meat every day. In the tests conducted prior to the experiment there was nothing unusual in the urine of these men. But within a few days of the start of the experiment, erythrocytes and albumin were detected in the urine of everyone of them.

It has been observed that reducing the proportion of proteins in the diet results in an increase in the physical and mental energy, a capacity to work for long duration without getting tired, and least danger of catching disease.

There is a relatively larger proportion of the amino acid methionine in meat. Many investigators believe that, if methionine is not metabolised properly in the body, the ultimate results are the development of atherosclerosis and the consequent increased risk of heart attack. Meat also contains large amounts of cholesterol. And vegetarians should keep it in mind that as milk is an animal product, it is not free from the above ingredient.

CARBOHYDRATES

Carbohydrates provide energy and heat to the body. Tubers, roots, pulses, milk, cereals, etc. are the main sources of carbohydrates.

There is no harm in the use of natural carbohydrates in their original forms. But the use of processed carbohydrates is not recommended. De-branned flour, polished rice, white flour, refined sugar, etc. are instances of such processed foods. Processing removes the fibres and roughage from the food. This results in insufficient elimination of wastes.Toxic substances consequently accumulate in the blood. Canned and bottled fruits, fruit juices, tomato ketchup, jams, jellies, instant gulabjamuns, rasagullas, ready-ground flours, cakes, chocolates, icecream, bread, biscuits, peppermint sweets and other similar processed carbohydrates cause plenty of damage to our health. As such foods are easily overeaten, the digestive organs are deal with heavy loads. The consequence is severe indigestion and obesity, resulting later everlasting diseased conditions like diabetes, or disorders of the joints.

Fats

Like carbohydrates, fats to perform the function of supplying heat and energy to the body. *Desi ghee* and oils are the main sources of fats for vegetarians.

Type of Fats

Fats are of two types—saturated and unsaturated. Regular use of saturated fats causes constriction and hardening of the arteries, which may result in hypertension, heart-attack and other related problems. Hence, one should minimise the intake of saturated fats, replacing them by unsaturated ones, if necessary.

Foods Having Saturated Fats

* Butter, *desi ghee*, vegetable ghee, coconut oil, palm oil.
* Cream, khoya, khoya-based preparations, sweets prepared in ghee and vegetable ghee, whole milk, whole-milk preparations (shreekhand, icecream, pedas, etc.).
* Cakes, biscuits, wafers, chocolates.
* Fat meat, oysters, fish, eggs.

Foods Having Unsaturated Fats

* Peanut oil, seasame oil, maize oil, soyabean oil, karadi oil, cottonseed oil, sunflower oil, and dishes prepared from these oils.

Quantities of Fats and Cholesterol in Food Items

Item	*Approximate Quantity*	*Weight (in Gms.)*	*Total Fats (in Gms.)*	*Satu-rated fats(in Gms.)*	*Unsaturated Fats*		*Choles-terol (in Mgs.)*
					Oleic Acid (in Gms.)	*Linoleic Acid (in Gms.)*	
1. Whole-Milk	1 Cup	240	8.5	4.9	3.6	—	27
2. Skimmed-Milk	1 Cup	240	—	—	—	—	7
3. Cake	1 Piece	50	14.0	2.0	—	0.5	45
4. Biscuit	1	35	6.5	2.3	3.4	0.8	17
5. Icecream	$\frac{1}{2}$ Cup	75	9.0	5.0	3.9	—	43
6. Butter	1 Teaspoon	5	4.0	2.3	1.2	—	12
7. Coconut Oil	1 Teaspoon	5	5.0	4.4	0.5	0.1	—
8. Karadi Oil	1 Teaspoon	5	5.0	0.4	1.0	3.6	—
9. Cottonseed Oil	1 Teaspoon	5	5.0	1.3	1.2	2.5	—
10. Peanut Oil	1 Teaspoon	5	5.0	0.9	1.6	2.5	—
11. Maize Oil	1 Teaspoon	5	5.0	0.5	1.8	2.7	—
12. Soyabin Oil	1 Teaspoon	5	5.0	0.8	1.6	2.6	—
13. Seasame Oil	1 Teaspoon	5	5.0	0.9	1.0	2.1	—
14. Liver	1 Oz	30	1.5	0.4	Trace	Trace	75
15. Bacon	1½ Oz	40	17.6	6.4	7.6	1.6	45
16. Egg	1	50	6.0	2.0	2.5	0.5	253
17. Oyster	1 Oz	30	1.9	0.6	1.0	0.3	45

Minerals and Vitamins

Our body requires only little quantities of these substances, but they are of great importance. They perform various important functions in the body. Vitamins are essential for the proper digestion and absorption of proteins, carbohydrates and fats, and the development of the quality of the body to protect itself against diseases. Various minerals are needed for the formation and functioning of the cells. These vital substances are necessary for the maintenance of health. Moreover, they are most essential in sickness. Deficiency of vitamins and minerals, may directly result in various kind of complications.

The reserves of the vitamins in the body get quickly depleted during an illness. Unbalanced diet, mental distress, pollution, smoking, addiction to drugs are other factors that destroy the vitamins in the body. The requirements of vitamins have increased to a great extent these days due to the mental stresses and worries which have become so common in modern hectic life. Unwholesome diet and the uninhibited use of medicines such as, antibiotics and cortisones also tend to reduce the reserves of vitamins in our bodies.

We need vitamins and minerals today as never before. Adequate quantities of these essential components of foods are available in uncooked foods, germinated grains and beans, as well as in vegetables, fruits and their juices.

Over-cooking destroys vitamins. The vitamins in fruits and vegetables are rapidly lost if they are not consumed immediately after cutting or peeling.

Though some experts say Vitamin B_{12} can be obtained only from meat. But meat can not be eaten raw, and cooking destroys most of the Vitamin B_{12} in it.

Please note that vitamins in natural foodstuffs are in easily digestible form, and so are quickly and completely assimilated in the body. On the other hand, experiments have decisively proved that the expected benefit is almost never afforded by the use of synthetic vitamins in the forms of tablets, pills, etc. In the same way, the body cannot satisfactorily utilise artificially synthesised or purified mineral salts. In nutshell, if the body lacks minerals, the deficiency cannot be made good by medicines or other synthetic items.

The ailments caused by deficiencies of vitamins and minerals, and also their functions and sources are given in the following tables:

Minerals

Mineral	*Daily Need of an Adult*	*Function*	*Sources*	*Probable Symptoms of Deficiency*
Sodium	2500 mg	Sodium is an important part of the extra-cellular fluids. 30 to 40 per cent sodium is present in the bones.	Milk, common salt, beetroots, carrots, radishes, *phanasi*, etc. contain sodium. It is also present in eggs, meat and fish.	Deficiency of sodium can cause headache, slower development of the body and disorders of the muscles, nausea.
Iron	10 mg	Nearly 70 per cent of the iron in the body is present in haemoglobin in red blood cells. 26 per cent iron is stored in the liver, spleen and bones. In the absence of iron, the cells cannot take up oxygen or eliminate carbon dioxide.	Mint and other green leafy vegetables, *methi*, seasame, millets, grams, green grams, black grams, soyabeans, dates, mangoes, etc. are good sources of iron. So are eggs, meat, animal livers, oysters, etc.	Anaemia is the main symptom of iron deficiency.
Sulphur	300 mg	Sulphur is a constituent of proteins, and some vitamins. It is also required for metabolic processes.	Beetroots, cabbage, garlic, onions; radishes, milk and meat are the sources of sulphur.	Some metabolic processes in the body are hindered by a deficiency of sulphur.

Minerals

Mineral	*Daily Need of an Adult*	*Function*	*Sources*	*Probable Symptoms of Deficiency*
Calcium	800 mg	99 per cent of calcium in the body is found in bones and teeth. It is also necessary for the transport of some substances into or out of cells.	*Methi*, drumsticks, and other green leafy vegetables, watermelons, millets, seasome, beetroots, figs, grapes, and black grams are good sources of calcium. Milk and milk products, some fish and oysters also contain plenty of calcium.	Deficiency of calcium weakens bones and teeth, and causes osteoporesis.
Chlorine	2000 mg	This element functions in association with sodium. It is one of the main constituents of extra cellular fluids. It activates certain enzymes. It is a constituent of the digestive juices of the stomach.	Common salt, milk, carrots, potatoes, spinach, cabbage, tomatoes, bananas, dates, etc. contain chlorine. Chlorine is also present in eggs, meat, and salt-water fish also.	Deficiency of chlorine weakens bones and stiffens joints.
Iodine	0.14 mg	It is a constituent of the secretion of the thyroid gland.	Iodine is present in seafoods and green vegetables.	Deficiency of iodine impairs the function of the thyroid gland, resulting in goitre.

Minerals

Mineral	*Daily Need of an Adult*	*Function*	*Sources*	*Probable Symptoms of Deficiency*
Phosphorus	800 mg	About 80 per cent of the phosphorus in the body is present in the bones and teeth. It is an important part of every cell. It helps to regulate the pH of the blood, and is necessary for the formation of substances like DNA, RNA, ATP, which are essential for life processes.	Cheese, milk, yeast, dry fruits, soyabeans, dates, carrots, guava, etc. are the sources of phosphorus. It is also present in eggs, meat and fish.	Deficiency of phosphorus causes weakening of the bones and teeth, and weight loss.
Potassium	2500 mg	Potassium is an important part of cellular fluid. It is required for the metabolism of carbohydrates and proteins. It helps in the regulation of the pH of the blood.	Plenty of potassium is supplied by milk, garlic, radishes, potatoes, fresh fruit and meat.	Deficiency of potassium may cause weakness of the muscles, even paralysis. It may also cause brittleness of the bones, sterility and heart ailments.
Magnesium	350 mg	Nearly 50 per cent magnesium is found in the bones and the remaining 50 per cent in the cells. Magnesium is necessary for the activation of many enzymes. Hence a large number of processes taking place in the body are dependent on magnesium.	Cereals, milk, green vegetables, dry fruit and meat contain magnesium.	Teeth, bones and muscles weaken due to the deficiency of magnesium. Insufficient supply of magnesium may even give rise to heart ailments.

Vitamin

Vitamin	Daily Need of an Adult	Function	Sources	Symptoms of Deficiency
Vitamin A	4000 to 5000 International units (I.U.)	This is necessary for the development and protection of certain cells in the body. It is essential for a healthy condition of the eyes. Night vision is also dependent on it. It is needed for the development of bones and formation of teeth.	Cheese, milk, butter, green leafy vegetables, cabbsages, carrots, red and yellow fruits and vegetables. Large amounts of Vitamin A are also found in fish liver oils.	Deficiency of Vitamin A slows down growth, causes dryness of skin and eyes, eventually leading to night blindness; deformation of bones and teeth may also result due to its deficiency.
Vitamin B This group of vitamins comprises eight vitamins: Vitamin B_1, Vitamin B_2, Niacin, Vitamin B_6, Pantothenic Acid, Biotin, Folcin and Vitamin B_{12}	0.5 to 5 mg of each vitamin of this group	This group of vitamins is necessary for the development of the body, appetite, healthy condition of eyes, nerves and skin, and for the prevention of anaemia.	Milk, wheat bran, yeast, germinated wheat, leafy vegetables, fresh vegetables and fruits, pulses, etc. are the usual sources. It is also present in meat (especially liver), fish, and eggs.	Deficiency of Vitamin B_1 causes beri-beri. Deficiency of Vitamin B_2 causes chaps on the skin around the eyes, nose and mouth. Niacin deficiency is responsible for pellagra and deterioration of nerves. Insufficient intake of Vitamin B_6 results in anaemia and skin diseases. Metabolic reactions are disrupted by a lack of pantothenic acid. The symptoms of deficiency of biotin or folcin resemble those caused by a lack of pantothenic acid. Deficiency of Vitamin B_{12} slows down growth and induces pernicious anaemia.

Vitamin

Vitamin	*Daily Need of an Adult*	*Function*	*Sources*	*Symptoms of Deficiency*
Vitamin C	45 mg	This is essential for the proper development of the body. It also helps the formation of bones and teeth. It helps various cells to cohere together, heals wounds, augments the resistance of the body to diseases, and is also a factor in the synthesis of steroid hormones in the body.	Sources of Vitamin C are sweetsour fruits, myrobalan, tomatoes, watermelons, pears, cabbages, pineapples, potatoes and green leafy vegetables.	Deficiency of Vitamin C causes scurvy, diseased conditions of teeth and gums, internal haemorrhage, osteoporesis, loss of weight, and in some cases, even sterility.
Vitamin D	300 to 400 I.U.	This is necessary for the development of the body. It plays an important part in the formation of bones and teeth.	Sunlight is the best source of Vitamin D. It is also present in milk, eggs and some fish liver oils.	Deficiency of Vitamin D causes osteoporesis. This leads to rickets in children.
Vitamin E	12 to 15 I.U.	This is important for the reproductive function. In addition, it strengthens the erythrocytes and prevents their fragmentation.	Germinated wheat, green leafy vegetables, vegetable oils, nuts, eggs and milk are sources of this vitamin.	Deficiency of this vitamin may cause sterility.
Vitamin K	1 to 2 mg	This is essential for the production of prothrombin, which is responsible for the clotting of blood.	It is found in green leafy vegetables, tomatoes, cauli-flower, wheat bran, soyabean oil, vegetable oils, and livers of animals.	Due to deficiency of this vitamin, prothrombin cannot be synthesized by the body. As a result blood fails to clot, and even minor cuts result in non-stop bleeding.

Balance of Acid and Alkali in Blood

The ratio of acids to alkalis in blood is generally 20 : 80. Maintenance of this ratio is very important. The body naturally works very hard to maintain this ratio.

After undergoing the full cycle of digestive and metabolic processes, some of our foods leave alkaline residue in the body, some others leave acidic residues. We may call such foods alkali-genic and acid-genic respectively. Generally, the acids produced by the metabolic activities, (such as uric acid, lactic acid, etc.) react with the alkalis in the blood, lymph, bile, etc. thus being neutralised and rendered innocuous. But if our diet is replete with acid-genic foods, the body cannot cope with all the resulting acids. When the acids accumulate in the blood, symptoms associated with acidic blood like headache, anorexia, insomnia, nervous tension, hyperacidity, coryza, fatigue, etc. come to surface.

Having more acid in blood is an abnormal condition that hinders the physical development of children and adolescents, causes degeneration in older people, and diminishes vitality. It causes difficulties in pregnancy and lactation. It is the origin of diseases like appendicitis, pneumonia, tuberculosis, cancer and measles.

All the toxic substances in the body are in the form of acids, and that in order to prevent or counteract the accumulation of acids in the body we must take food that is mainly alkali-genic.

One must know that what food will result in the generation of how much alkalinity or acidity in the body.

Alkali-Genic Foods		**Acid-Genic Foods**	
Food	*Alkali-genic effect in per cent*	*Food*	*Acid-genic effect in per cent*
Milk and Milk Products:			
Human Milk	2.25	**Food of Animal Origin (Excluding milk):**	
Cow's Milk	1.69		
Butter Milk	1.31		
Goat's Milk	0.25	Beef	38.61
Skimmed Milk	4.89	Chicken	24.32
Cream	2.66	Goat's Flesh	20.30
Fruits:		Fish	19.52
		Pork	12.47
Apricots (fresh)	4.79	Yolk of Egg	51.83
Bananas	4.38	White of Egg	8.27
Pomegranates	4.15	Eggs	11.61
Coconuts	4.09		
Pineapples	3.59	**Milk Products:**	
Pears	3.26		
Watermelons	1.83		
Apples	1.38	Cheese	17.49
Figs (fresh)	27.81	Butter	4.33
Raisins	15.10		
Grapes	7.15		
Sugarcane	14.57	**Cereals:**	
Tomatoes	13.67		
Lemons	9.90	Cake	12.31
Oranges	9.61	Bread	10.99
Plums	5.80	Barley	10.58
Dates	5.50	White Flour (wheat)	8.32
Peaches	5.40	Maize	5.37
Vegetables, Tubers and Roots:		Wheat	2.66
		Rice (polished)	17.96
Potatoes	5.90	Rice (manually de-husked)	3.68
Peas (fresh)	5.15		
Cabbage	4.02	**Nuts:**	
Cauliflower	3.04		
Onions	1.09	Almonds	2.19
Pumpkin	0.28	Peanuts	16.39
Spinach	28.01	Walnuts	9.22
Suva Plants	18.36		
Leafy Salad Plants	14.12		
Cucumbers	13.50	**Pulses and Legumes:**	
Beetroots	11.37		
Turnips	10.80		
Sweet Potatoes (years)	10.31	All pulses and legumes	
Radishes	6.05	Highly acid-genic	

After going through the table, you would have noticed that meat, fish, eggs and pulses are highly acid-genic. Wholemeal wheat flour, manually dehusked unpolished rice, and such other cereals in their more or less natural forms are only mildly acid-genic, but processing or refining them makes them much more acidic in effect. All vegetables, tubers, roots and fruits are alkali-genic. Green leafy vegetables are more alkali-genic than any other food item.

Now let us think about our usual daily fare in the context of this table. For breakfast we usually take milk, tea, coffee, buns, chiwda, *matthi*, biscuits, etc. All these foods are acid-genic. Dal, rice and chapaties, which are the mainstays of the mid-day meal, are also highly acid-genic. Only the vegetables are alkali-genic. But even in their case the alkalis have been rendered ineffective by oxidation during the process of cooking. Refreshments in the afternoon also consist of tea and fried preparations, or in some cases sweets, sandwiches, idlis, dosas, etc. Most of these are again acid-forming. Rice, dal, curry, khichdi which comprise the usual evening meal are all acid genic foods. The enormous amounts of the alkalis stored in the body which are wasted in counteracting this onslaught of acids can only be conjectured. We are not habitual of regularly taking alkali-genic foods like fruits. And we have not realized the importance of uncooked vegetables at all. Due to this we regularly fall victim to diseases.

One can easily maintain a balance between the acids and alkalis in the body by a judicious combination of various unprocessed cereals, raw vegetables, fruits and nuts in our daily diet and thus keep diseases at bay. Not only do the alkalis in such foods neutralize the acids in other foods, but they also help in extracting the acids and toxins accumulated in the cells of the body, and ejecting them from the system. These qualities make a diet made up of alkali-genic components pure and wholesome.

The food consisting of dead matter cannot enliven the body. Cooking our food, and thus rendering it lifeless, has become an established convention. Wild animals survive on uncooked food, and though domesticated animals like dogs, cats and cows may find cooked food acceptable, but if given a free choice they would always like to have raw uncooked food.

In human body, the cells die, and are replaced by new ones. These processes of regeneration require vitamins, mineral salts and enzymes. Vitamins and enzymes are also necessary for the digestion and assimilation of proteins, carbohydrates, fats, etc. These enzymes and some of the vitamins are destroyed by heat. Hence cooked food does not contain them in adequate amounts.

Meals prepared to please only the taste buds are scarcely suitable for the nutrition of the body. Spices may vastly improve the taste of foods, so that it can be consumed with relish, but that is hardly the only or the main purpose of taking food. We eat to live, and do not—or should not—live to eat. And we need not disregard taste completely: proper combinations of the natural flavours can make even uncooked foods tasty and appetising, some people may develop taste for such kinds of food after some time.

Over-cooking not only destroys vitamins and enzymes in the foods, but also results in degradation of their nutritive value. Proteins in foods are coagulated and hardened by cooking. Such coagulated proteins are not digested, but decay in the digestive tract. Cooking also makes carbohydrates less easy to digest. As a result, they are not absorbed completely in the intestines. Thus, in terms of nutrients our cooked foods are comparatively almost valueless. A healthy person may still be able to extract the residual nutrients from them, but this is hardly possible for one who is ill and require them very badly.

An expert says that cooked food is the oldest addiction of mankind. 95 per cent of physical and mental disorders are the products of such lifeless food.

If we choose right food combinations, only then we can ensure proper digestion. If the rules are violated, even good nutritious food may produce toxic materials as a result of decomposition in the digestive tract. For example, there is no enzyme in the stomach which can digest carbohydrates. Carbohydrates are digested either in the mouth or in the small intestine. On the other hand, the digestion of proteins takes place in the stomach. Let us consider a meal that contains large quantities of both carbohydrates and proteins. If it is masticated properly, the enzymes in the saliva in the mouth carry out partial digestion of the carbohydrates. But if the food is swallowed without adequate mastication, the carbohydrates will remain undigested in the stomach while the proteins are being digested. They will, therefore, decay and produce toxic materials. For example, if a morsel of chapati is chewed well, the carbohydrates in it will be converted into sugars, imparting a sweet taste to the morsel.

These sugars are absorbed directly into the blood stream as soon as they reach the stomach. Now if the chapaties are not chewed properly, the carbohydrates are in a completely undigested condition, with the result that they start decaying in the stomach. An important point to be noted is that the enzymes in the saliva can act only in an alkaline medium. If sour chutneys or pickles are taken along with a morsel of the chapati, or if the vegetable or dal taken with the chapati contain limes, tomatoes, tamarind or similar sources of acids, the enzymes in the saliva get de-activated, and therefore completely undigested carbohydrates find their way into the stomach. It is, therefore, advisable not to take chapaties and sour foods simultaneously. This combination will produce toxic substances in the body.

The germination of grain and pulses results in a vast increase in their nutritive contents. In uncooked germinated seeds, there is an increase up to 600 per cent in the amounts of thiamin (Vitamin B_1), pantothenic acid, niacin, etc. and that too in a natural, live form. The number of yeast cells, so useful to the body, increases by 6 thousand million. Lactation in nursing mothers increases considerably by the consumption of germinated cereals and pulses, hence they may feed infant without facing insufficient lactation problem.

This belief that raw food is indigestible, and will cause heaviness in the belly, stomach ache or gas, is erroneous. It has been established by experiments that cooked foods require five to six hours for complete digestion, while raw foods need only three to four hours. Fruit and vegetable juices are digested, and begin to get absorbed, in only twenty-five to thirty minutes. Thus uncooked food, and especially uncooked liquid food, gives rest to the digestive organs. The valuable energy of the body is not wasted in useless, futile attempts at digesting the indigestible, and thus becomes available for healing and regeneration.

By proper nutrition it is possible to keep the human body, alive and active for long time.

Rules for Selection of Food Combinations

* Proteins in large amounts should not be taken simultaneously with large amounts of fats (e.g., dal and ghee), because these two types of foods are digested in different parts of the digestive tract.
* The foods containing proteins should not be ingested with sour fruits. For instance, if lemon juice or tomatoes are added to dal, the acids in these fruits cause a diminution in the secretion of digestive juices, rendering digestion less efficient.
* Large amounts of proteins and large amounts of carbohydrates should not be taken at the same time.
* Carbohydrates should not be mixed with sour foods.

People with weaker constitution or weaker digestive powers should follow these rules strictly. People in robust health may not suffer any serious ill effects by ingesting foods in improper combinations. It is also a fact that nature itself has combined carbohydrates and proteins, or proteins and fats, together in many foods; it is not possible to effect a separation of these constituents.

An Ideal Diet Schedule

Early morning: Juice of one lemon or half a lemon mixed in a glass of water. People suffering from a cold should take the juice in warm water. No sugar, salt or honey should be mixed.

Breakfast: Fruits or fruit juice; bananas, dates, raisins, dry fruit and similar nutritious foods may also be consumed.

Lunch: Have half a cup of the uncooked juice of leafy vegetables, or a cup of soup of such vegetables. This can be followed by some germinated pulses, some raw vegetables, and if desired, some sweet-sour fruits, but do not forget masticate well. The meal may be concluded with wheat chapaties and boiled vegetables. Rice can be substituted for the chapaties. Occasionally, the meal may be ended with buttermilk.

4.00 to 5.00 in the evening: Fruits, or fruit juice.

Dinner: Same as lunch, except that the uncooked juice of vegetables should be omitted. The chapaties may be made from other cereals. People endowed with robust health and strong digestion may occasionally even take khichdi; or a small bowl of dal with rice at lunch or dinner time.

Do not forget that the bran should not be separated from the wheat flour. Manually de-husked rice only should be used, not polished rice. No sour ingredients like tomatoes, tamarind, etc. should be added to vegetables or dal, and a minimum amount of salt should be added to them. Salt should never be added to buttermilk, or sprinkled on fruits or salad.

Some Suggestions

* Avoid eating or drinking anything that is too hot or too cold, the temperature of any food should be around 37°C (98.6°F), the temperature of the body. The enzymes in the mouth and the stomach act best at such temperatures.
* Avoid food when you are physically or mentally tense, If the body or the mind is exhausted or tense, the secretion of the digestive juices will not be upto the mark.
* Consider first the wholesomeness (or otherwise) of food combinations, even alkali-genic and nutritious foods, when taken without regard to the rules of

food combinations, can generate toxins in the body to pave way for diseases.

* Avoid drinking water with meals because water requires only ten minutes to be absorbed from the stomach, and in the process it carries the enzymes away. This reduces the efficiency of the digestive process, which may result in the loss of appetite. There is no harm in drinking water fifteen minutes before a meal, half an hour after taking fruits, and two hours after a meal.
* Always chew your food well, because thorough chewing mixes saliva with the food. Digestion starts off in the mouth itself with the action of the enzymes present in the saliva. Moreover, well-chewed food is easily digested in the system.
* Have only one meal, or take only fruits, one day every week, because giving occasional rest to the stomach is as necessary as giving it is usual assignment of digestion, for maintaining its efficiency. Moreover, when the body is not occupied in the task of digestion, it is free to tackle the poisons that have been accumulated in it, and if that is done efficiently then diseases would not be able to launch attack.
* Avoid any kind of food while suffering from fever or any other ailment. You must be aware of this fact that we never feel hunger when we are indisposed, and actually feel averse to taking any food. During an illness, the secretion of digestive juices is greatly reduced. As a result, the digestive processes are almost at a standstill, in such a condition food should be avoided to your own good.
* Avoid overeating, because it is always harmful. The stomach is a flexible bag made up of muscles. Its rhythmic contractions and expansions are responsible for the efficient mixing of digestive juices and enzymes with food. These movements are hindered if the bag is stuffed up with excessive food. The enzymes are not mixed properly with the food, which begins to decay. Most people fail to exercise discretion in the

amount of food they take. They live to eat, not eat to live. Overeating makes one lethargic and dull. There is a constant feeling of thirst. With time the belly gets enlarged, and one falls victim to disorders of the digestive system. To keep healthy it is necessary at all times to remain slightly hungry. And remember that excess of everything is harmful whether it is food, medicine, or anything.

* Do not eat if you are not hungry, animals would eat without hunger, due to this they are not subject to the ailments which man invites by overburdening the digestion. When really hungry, we relish even the most insipid and unappetising foods. Moreover in such condition we do not hesitate more than our requirement.

* You should rest for a while after meals, because the blood vessels of the stomach dilate just after meals. This stimulates the secretion of enzymes, and thus helps digestion. If work requiring any kind of physical or mental exertion is taken up just after a meal, blood will be diverted from the stomach to other parts of the body like the hand, feet or brain, slowing down digestion process.

Modern medicine measures food value in terms of calorics. Though energy is something fundamental to the organism and can be enhanced because of the ability of the system to absorb it from the foodstuffs consumed, but if the foodstuffs lack the important elements, then the vital force of body is not enhanced. Hence, the balanced diet and right combination is essential to remain healthy and disease-free.

CHAPTER 3

Juices

The best food is the one which is consumed in the same form in which nature provides it. Now you know that alkali-genic foods, extract the toxic substances accumulated in the cells of the body and help in their elimination. And this is why such foods are considered to be purifying foods. Seventy-five per cent of the diet of a patient should consist of alkaline substances.

It is said that well-chewed vegetables and fruits can supply all the necessary minerals and vitamins equally well, but no one can eat a enough raw vegetables and fruits, if they have to be thoroughly chewed. For instance, one can eat a tomato or two at a time, no more. But it would, be quite easy to drink the juice of eight or ten tomatoes. It must also be remembered that, even if fruits and vegetables are well chewed, a large amount of fibres and woody particles will reach the stomach, loading the stomach and slowing down digestion. Hence, when the digestive system is not to be overburdened, and, at the same time, fasting is not desirable for some reason, a juice diet, consisting of juices of vegetables and fruits, becomes a necessity.

Alkali-genic diet, rich in minerals, is all the more necessary in sickness. Sickness is rooted in acids accumulated in the body. To neutralise and deactivate these acids, one must take food which can supply plenty of alkalis. This purpose can be better served by a liquid diet like juice.

For the best supply of alkalis to the body, there is nothing that is better than a diet of juices. Such a diet also provides sufficient vitamins and enzymes that augment the resistive and healing powers of the systems of the body.

Many experts say that fruit and vegetable juices must not be mixed, but must always be taken separately.

Artificial foods available in food stores are responsible for many of the disorders that cause serious trouble for the users. Hence, canned or bottled juices are entirely worthless for health, as all the active constituents useful for fighting diseases or promoting health have been destroyed by the processing and prolonged storage. Moreover, harmful chemicals have been added to the juices as preservatives. No one should allow himself to be misguided by the labels declaring that the cans or bottles contain 'fresh juice'. Moreover, most of them are synthetic, hence, one should avoid them.

Always consume juice while fresh. This is especially important when the purpose is that of healing or prevention of disease. The vitamins in raw uncooked foods are very sensitive to the oxygen of the air. If carrots, for example, are cut or shredded and then left for some time, most of their Vitamin A content gets destroyed by oxidation within 20 to 25 minutes. In the same way, lemons, oranges, apples, and similar fruits lose about 50 per cent of their Vitamin C content in only one month, during storage. If the vitamins in uncut fruits and vegetables are destroyed so easily, it is obvious that the vitamins in their juices must get destroyed much more quickly. The juices, therefore, must be taken immediately as soon as they are extracted. The juices must not be gulped down, but sipped slowly, so as to give saliva a chance to mix with them and begin the process of the digestion of the carbohydrates before its journey to the stomach.

CHAPTER 4

Exercises for Strong Body

A person falls sick when his defences are down. The vital force of our body keeps us alive, acting as a bulwark against decay and diseases. The vital force is storehouse of our physical strength. Hence, for maintenance of perfect health, exercise is no less important than diet. The reason why the people belonging to old times were healthier and stronger than we are is that they led comparatively much more strenuous lives. Today's mechanization has made us less active.

The Effect of Exercise on Various Organs and Systems

The skin: During exercise the pores of the skin open up. The result is a healthier skin, because of more efficient disposal of dirt and waste material.

Temperature of the body: During exercise the temperature of the body rises significantly. This promotes the burning up of the toxic substances in the body.

The musculature: Muscles are strengthened by regular exercise, it develops them and increases their efficiency. Stronger muscles lend better support to the joints.

The respiratory system: Because of exercise the breathing becomes not only more rapid, but also deeper, thus making increased quantities of oxygen available for the body cells.

The digestive system: Secretion of the digestive juices is stimulated by exercise. Thus digestion becomes more efficient. Exercises also stimulate the intestinal movements, resulting in more effective elimination of wastes in the form of bowels and urine.

Heart and circulatory system: The muscles of heart get stronger and more capable by regular exercise. The heart-beats of an athlete do not increase appreciably even when doing something requiring physical exertion, and revert very soon to the normal rate afterwards. In contrast, even a little exertion sends the pulse rate of a sedentary individual shooting up, and it takes time for the heart to settle down to its normal rate of beating. The blood vessels dilate during exercise, and so more blood reaches the muscles. It has been found that during vigorous or rapid exercise, the blood circulation in certain muscles and organs increases 25 to 30 times, thus supplying the muscles and organs with more oxygen and a larger number of red blood corpuscles.

In nutshell, all the systems of the body derive tremendous benefits from exercise. Each one of us should set aside a minimum period of 30 to 40 minutes every day in the morning for exercise, we spend time in various activities, why not spend a small part of the day on our bodies?

For perfect health, we must two type of exercises: The Yogic Aasanas and the exercises involving rapid movements, such as jogging or swimming. Yogic aasanas tone up the internal organs of the body by subjecting them to contractions and dilations. Exercises involving rapid movements are beneficial for the heart and the blood vessels.

YOGAASANAS

Here is an ideal programme of yogic aasanas for the stimulation of all the organs and systems.

Trikonaasana

* Stand upright, planting the feet a foot and a half apart. Extend the arms horizontally outward, at the level

of the shoulders. Now bend towards the right at the waist, and try to touch the right foot, keeping the left arm vertical in the direction opposite to that of the right arm. Hold this position for some time, and resume the initial position. Execute a similar movement on the left side.

* Repeat this movement six times on each side.

Benefits

* This aasana stretches the spine laterally.
* The spleen and the liver are strengthened by contractions and dilations.

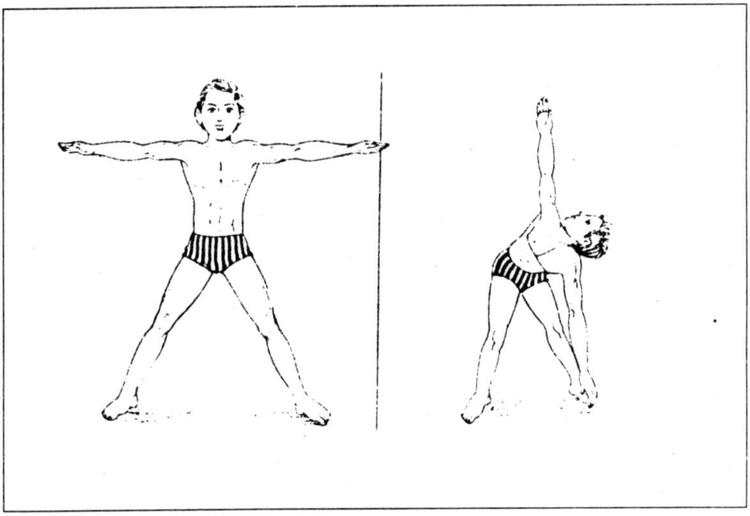

Fig. 1: Trikonaasana

Katimanthna

* Stand upright, planting the feet about a foot and a half apart. Extend the arms horizontally outwards at the level of the shoulders. Now, without changing positions of the feet, turn the torso round towards the left, and then towards the right.

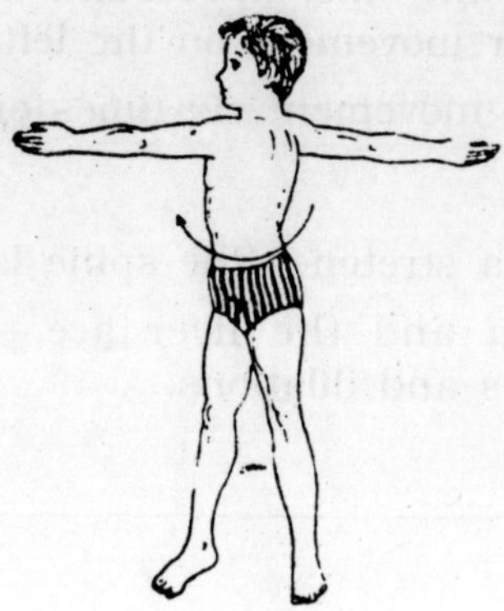

Fig. 2: Katimanthna

* Repeat the movement 6 times on each side.

Benefits

* This aasana keeps the spine flexible by subjecting it to rotatory movement.

Paschimottanaasna

* Sit on the floor and extend the two legs forward, parallel to and touching each other. Extend the arms forward horizontally at the level of the shoulders. Bend slowly forward, and try to touch the feet with the hands. Hold this position for some time, and resume the initial position.

Benefits

* This aasana flexes the spine forward.
* This aasana tightens the muscles of the organs in the abdomen, thus increasing their efficiency.
* The muscles of the back become flexible, and the waist becomes less rigid.

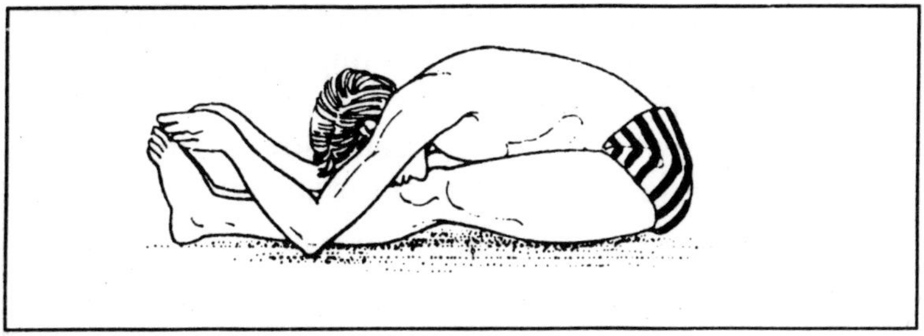

Fig. 3: Paschimottanaasna

A Word of Caution

* Hernia patient must be very careful while performing this aasana.

* This aasana is contra-indicated during pregnancy.

Ardhamatsyendraasna

* Sit down on the floor with the heel of the left foot touching the perineum. Place the right foot on the left of the left knee. Hold the big toe on the right foot with the

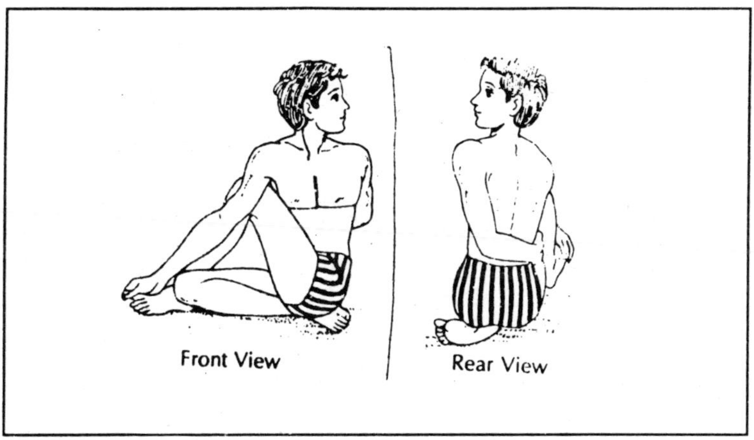

Fig. 4: Ardhamatsyendraasna

left hand, and with the right forearm placed horizontally in contact with the back, turn the upper part of the torso towards the right. Now carry out the same procedure on the other side, with the right heel at the perineum, the left foot placed on the right of the right knee.

* Repeat 6 times alternately for each side.

Benefits

* In this aasana, the vertebrae are made to rotate, thus helping to keep the spine flexible and elastic.

Matsyaasna

* Sit on the floor with the legs crossed. Incline the torso gradually backwards till it rests on the floor. Now grasp the big toes of the feet by the two hands, and bend the neck backwards. Take deep, slow breaths. In the final stage of the aasana, the weight of the torso is to be supported only by the head, the elbows and the buttocks.

Duration

* This aasana should be held initially for half a minute, and its duration should be gradually increased to two minutes.

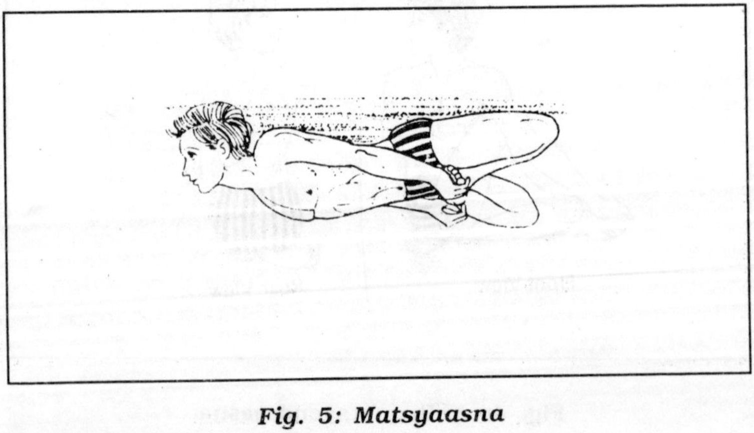

Fig. 5: Matsyaasna

Benefits

* The spine becomes supple and flexible.
* The respiratory system works more efficiently.

Dhanuraasna

* Lie face down on the floor. Raise the feet by bending the legs at the knees. Stretch the arms backwards to hold of the legs slightly above the ankles as shown in the figure. Raise the upper part of the torso, and the thighs, away from the floor, leaving only the pelvic region resting on the floor. Hold this position for some time, then resume the initial position.

* Perform this aasana 3 times.

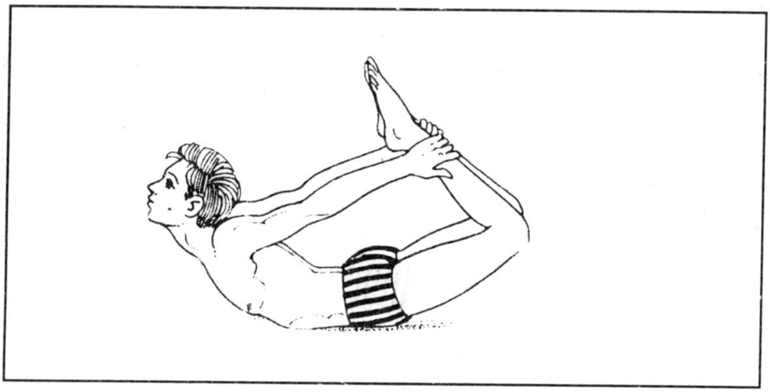

Fig. 6: Dhanuraasna

Benefits

* This aasana flexes the spine backwards.
* The organs in the abdomen are stretched.
* The muscles of the back and the waist become stronger.

Sarvaangaasna

* Lie down face up on the floor. Raise the legs slowly, keeping them straight at the knees. Follow this movement

by a gradual raising of the lower parts of the torso. Support the back with the palms, with the elbows resting on the floor. On completion of this movement, only the head, the nape, and the arms from the shoulders to the elbows will rest on the floor, the rest of the body will be straight and vertical.

Duration

* Hold this position for half a minute initially. Increase the duration gradually to two minutes.

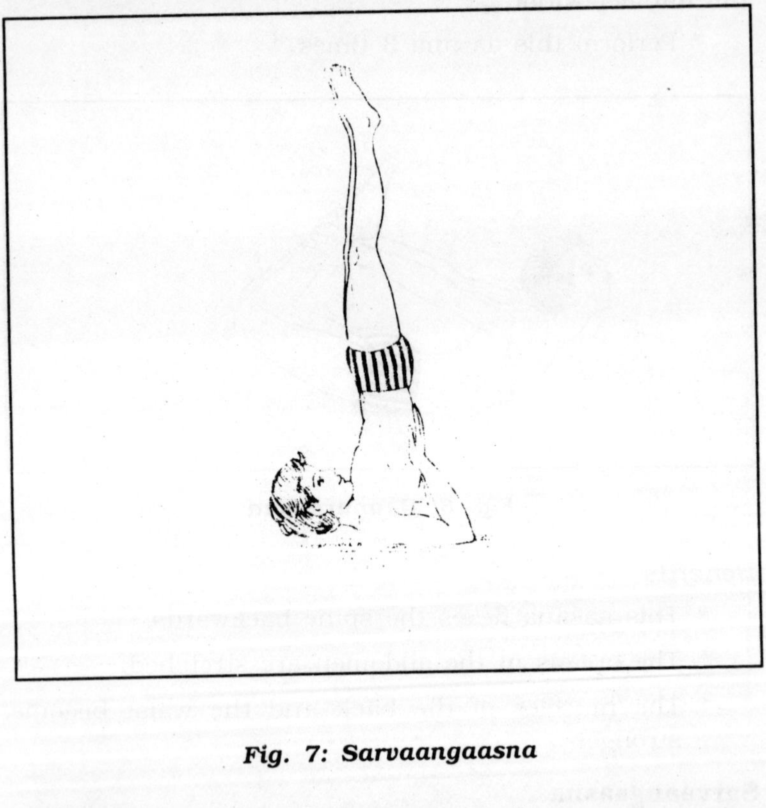

Fig. 7: Sarvaangaasna

Benefits

* The blood flows to the head and the upper part of the torso, nourishing these parts.

* The thyroid and the parathyroid glands are exercised by compression.

A Word of Caution

Those suffering from hypertension or heart ailments should avoid this aasana.

Sheershaasana

* In this aasana the body has to be inverted and balanced on the head. In the beginning, the position should be assumed with somebody's help, or by using a wall for support while going through the initial stages. Later on one should develop the ability of assuming and holding the position without help or support.

Duration

* This aasana should be held for half a minute initially, and its duration should be gradually increased to two minutes.

Benefits

* This aasana promotes circulation in the upper parts of the body, and keeps them healthy.

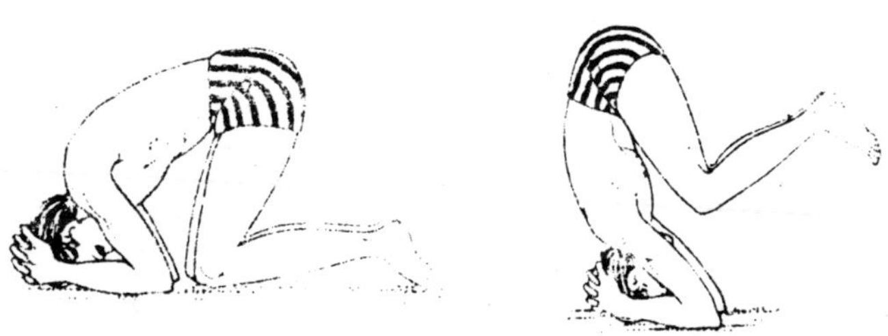

Step–1 Step-2

Fig. 8: Sheershasana

A Word of Caution

People suffering from hypertension or heart diseases must not perform this aasana.

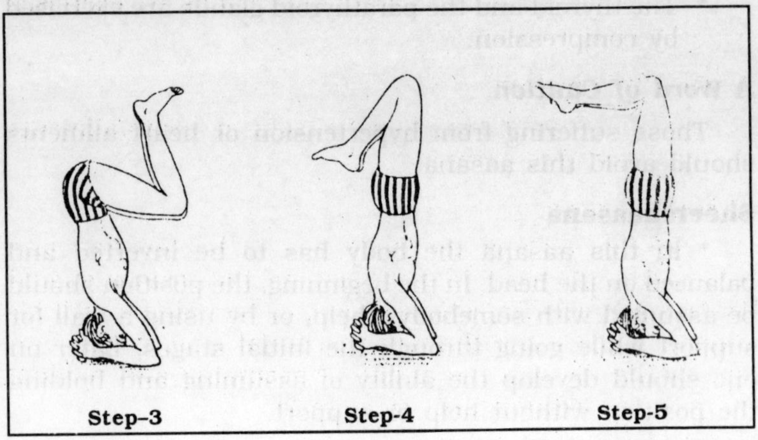

Fig. 9

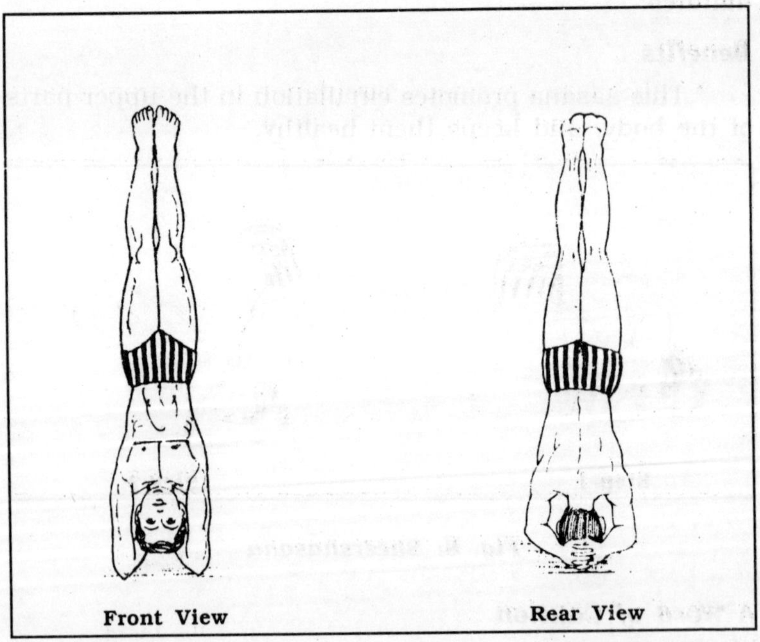

Fig. 10

* The eyes should be kept closed during performing this aasana.

Shavaasna

* This aasana must follow the preceding eight aasnas, or any other exercise.

* This aasana is also known as 'Mritasana'. Both the names signify the simulation of a deadbody. In this aasna, an attempt is made to dissociate the mind from the body. For getting maximum rest in the minimum time, there is nothing better than the Shavaasna. The Shavaasna is worldwide acknowledged for relieving the psychological tensions generated by hectic and competitive life of modern times.

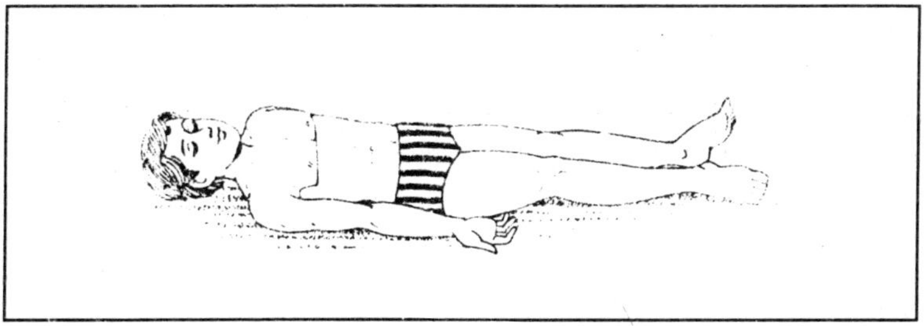

Fig. 11: Shavaasana

The Three Stages

First stage: Lie face up on the floor without a pillow. Keep the arms and legs relaxed in convenient positions. Now relax the muscles of the body, making a conscious attempt to relax each of the muscles of the body. Begin with the muscles of the legs. Relax and loosen them as much as you can. Then successively relax the muscles of the thighs, lower torso, upper torso, arms, neck and face. The body should seem lifeless to an onlooker.

Second stage: After relaxing all the muscles, turn your attention to your breathing. Inhale extremely slowly, and release the breath equally slowly. Gradually, slow down the breathing action to such an extent that an onlooker may not be able to detect it.

Third stage: The third stage of the Shavaasna is of great importance. But it is somewhat difficult and gaining proficiency in it requires some practice and time.

* The aim in this stage is to slow down the activity of the mind to a great extent. The ideal state of the mind aimed at in this aasna is a complete cessation of thought; but this state is not attainable by all. However, most of the desired benefit can be obtained if the mind can be induced to hold benign, religious positive thoughts.

Try to visualize a religious symbol at the point of the forehead between the two eyebrows, and concentrate the mind on it. Or go on repeating mentally a religious verse or a name of God. Initially, you will find that the mind wanders off to mundane thoughts. As soon as you become aware that this has happened, concentrate anew on the symbol, or the repetition.

Duration

* Holding this aasana for ten to fifteen minutes bring a sense of indescribable, restfulness, contentment and peace.

EXERCISE INVOLVING RAPID MOVEMENTS

In modern times the majority of people suffering from heart ailments is increasing by leaps and bounds. Heart disease is the main culprit in most of the deaths in urban areas. Therefore exercises for strengthening the heart—and thus reducing the probability of heart disease should be undertaken seriously and immediately. The heart can be strengthened and made more efficient by exercises involving rapid and continuous movements for at least fifteen minutes, so that the rate of heart-beats is increased. and remains high for some time. Exercises serving this purpose include rapid walking, jogging, swimming and cycling.

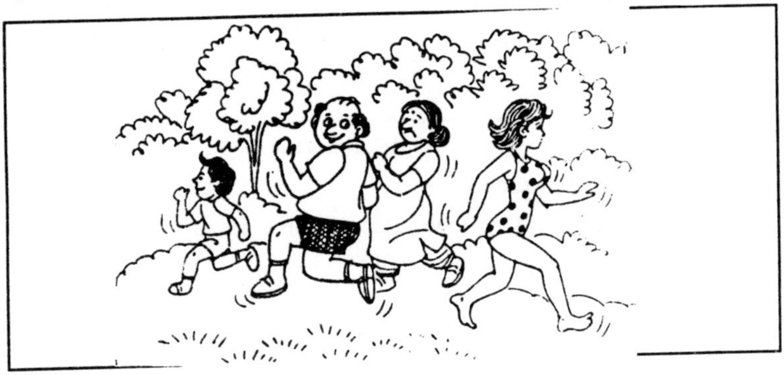

Fig. 12: Exercise Involving Rapid Movements

How to Begin?

Before starting a programme of exercises, you must ascertain your normal, resting pulse-rate. Before you get up in the morning, place your fingers on one of the locations indicated by circles in Figure 12.

* On the wrist near the base of the thumb.

or *On the neck beside the Adam's Apple.

If you would place your fingers correctly on the arteries, you will be able to feel the pulses as the heart forces the blood through them. Count the number of pulses in one minute, and note down in a table, as shown below:

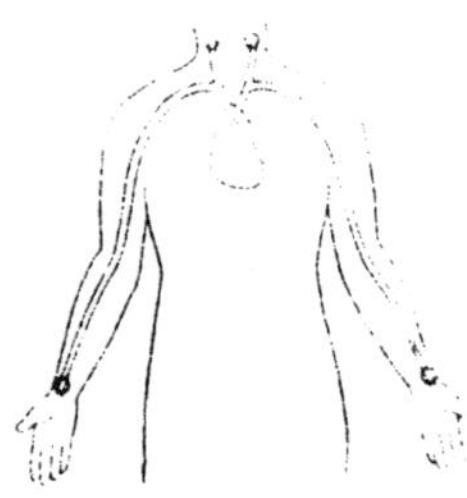

Fig. 13

	Date	Pulse-rate per minute
1		
2		

Preserve the paper for future use.

Preparatory Programme

One must start preparations fifteen days prior to a programme of exercises for increasing the efficiency of the heart. In the preparatory stage you must carry on activities that raise your pulse rate to the range described as the 'warm-up zone'.

Pluse Rate in the Warm-up Zone

Age (Years)	*Pulse-rate in Warm-up Zone (per minute*
30-34	116-126
35-39	112-122
40-44	108-118
45-49	104-114
50-54	100-110
55-59	96-106
60-64	92-102
65 and over	86-96

For example, the appropriate pulse rate in the warm-up zone for a person who is 30-34 years old is 116 to 126 pulses per minute.

Find out a way of accommodating a 15 minute period of exercise in your daily routine: (Of course, this means that you will have to walk back the same distance again in the evening. But this only means additional benefit.) Or you can walk when you take your child to school, or when you go for shopping. Or you can go for a brisk walk in the early morning.

* Go for rapid walk in the early morning.

* Try to walk at least 2 kilometres in day time.

For two weeks, carry on above mentioned activities. Remember that the activity should be brisk enough to raise your pulse rate to the warm-up zone (you will have to determine your pulse-rate to ascertain this) and to maintain it at that rate for some time after the cessation of the activity (for which you will have to determine the pulse rate 5 to 7 minutes after cessation of the activity).

This is just a preparatory stage of the programme of exercises, not the programme itself. During this stage the muscles and the joints begin to get accustomed to brisk activity, decreasing the possibility of pain in the muscles and joints then the main programme is implemented. Moreover, this stage helps you to make sure that you can undertake a programme of strenuous exercises without any problem.

The Main Programme

The main programme should be undertaken after the preparatory programme of two weeks as mentioned earlier.

Age (Years)	*Target Zone Pulse-rate*	*Danger Zone Pulse-rate*
30-34	136-164	Exceeding 164
35-39	132-160	Exceeding 160
40-44	128-156	Exceeding 156
45-49	124-152	Exceeding 152
50-54	120-146	Exceeding 146
55-59	116-140	Exceeding 140
60-64	112-136	Exceeding 136
65 and over	106-130	Exceeding 130

For example, the desirable pulse-rate in the target zone for a person who is 30-34 years old is 136 to 156 pulses per minute.

The heart will derive tremendous benefit and its efficiency and endurance will be increased, only if the exercises raise the pulse-rate to the target zone (and the pulse-rate remains higher than normal for a few minutes afterwards).

Start an activity or an exercise that suits you and that is brisk enough to raise your pulse rate to the target zone. Young people will notice that they need exercises involving more rapid movements (jogging, swimming, etc.) to raise their pulse-rates suitably, whereas older persons would need less strenuous exercises (walking, etc.). However, whatever your age, after about a month you will find that you need more rapid movements to raise the pulse-rate to the target zone. This is a clear indication that the heart has become more efficient, and is able to cope with increase in the oxygen demand of the body with a smaller number of beats.

Some Suggestions

* The daily period of exercises should be about 40 minutes.

* The initial 6-10 minutes should be spent in activity which raises the pulse-rate to the warm-up zone. During this period, the muscles limber up and the blood vessels begin to dilate.

* The next 15-20 minutes should be spent in the main activity which causes the pulse-rate to touch the target zone.

* The activity should not be discontinued abruptly after 15-20 minutes of strenuous exercise, but should change over to less strenuous activity for about five minutes. It is highly important that the activity should be gradually slackened, and then stopped. During the period of strenuous activity, the heart pumps the blood rapidly into the arteries. At the same time, due to the pressure on the veins caused by the contraction of the muscles, the blood returns with equal rapidity to the heart. Now, if the activity is stopped suddenly, the contraction of the muscles ceases, but the rate of heart-beats does not decrease immediately. This results in an accumulation of blood in the limbs, and so the flow of blood to the brain is decreased. This may result in giddiness or even temporary unconsciousness.

* Remember that exercise should be rapid and strenuous enough to raise the pulse-rate to the target zone if it is to benefit the heart. But it is necessary to see that the pulse-rate does not touch the danger zone.

* After the exercises, do not take a hot-water bath, a sauna bath or a steam-bath. Only cold-water bath is suitable after exercise.

* It is essential that one should be regular in the programme of exercises. Exercises must be performed daily, or at least every alternate day. Performing them only once or twice a week, or at irregular intervals, cannot yield the expected result.

* Note down your resting pulse-rate—before leaving the bed in the morning—two months after starting the programme of exercise as described above. Compare it with the prior rate. The rate will show a dramatic decrease. This is decisive evidence that the efficiency of the heart has improved.

If the heart has been made more efficient by a programme of regular exercises involving rapid movements, the danger of a heart-attack is almost nil.

In this chapter you have got information about yogic aasnas and exercise involving rapid movements. Half an hour has to be allotted every day to each of these types. Those for whom it is possible to do this should do the yogasnas first, and then the latter type of exercises. Those who cannot spare so much time daily must give only half an hour a day to exercise, performing each type of exercise on alternate days.

'Suryanamaskara', is such an exercise which combines the benefits of both these types of exercises up to an extent.

Surya Namaskar

How to perform Surya Namaskar.

* This exercise should be performed preferably in the open, in the sunlight of early morning.

If a person cannot undertake other exercises, he should perform suryanamaskar 10 to 15 minutes a day. The performing them should be progressively increased. If suryanamaskaras is performed in open air in the mild sunlight of the early morning, one derives the benefits of sun bath in addition to the benefits of the suryanamaskara itself.

Namaskaaraasna

Position 1

Exhale and fold your hands in front of your chest in the gesture of a prayer, bringing your awareness to the heart centre or Sun God.

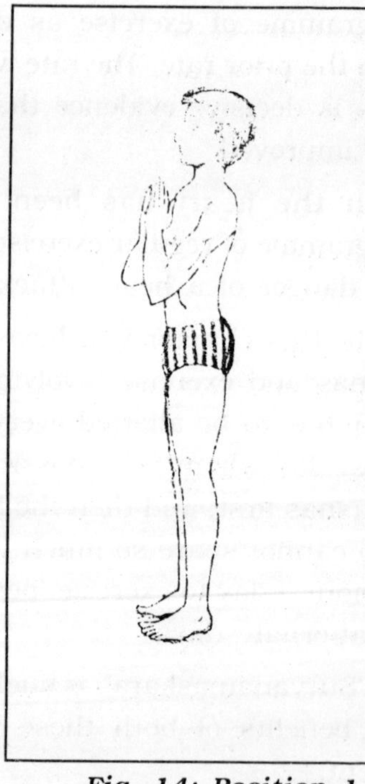

Fig. 14: Position 1

Position 2

Inhale deeply and raise your hands up and stretch backwards with your eyes open. Bringing your awareness to the throat centre. You may not be able to bend back very far initially, so go as far as you can without straining yourself. To avoid giddiness, keep your eyes open, and focused at a fix point.

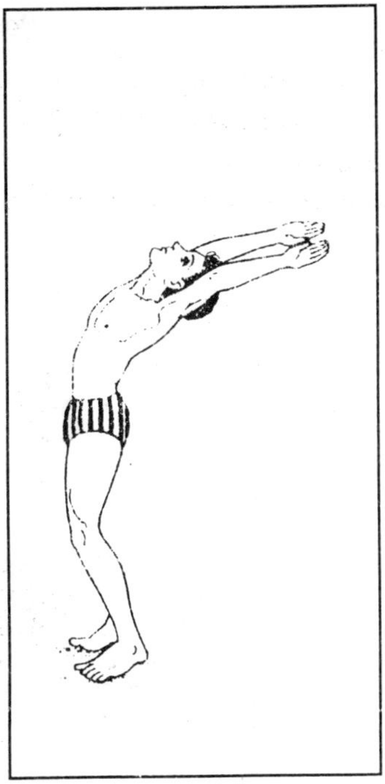

Fig. 15: Position 2

Position 3

Exhale and bend down completely to touch the ground with the palms of your hand. If you cannot bend completely, bend as far as possible and then bend your knees to rest your palms on the ground. Bring your awareness to the root of the spine.

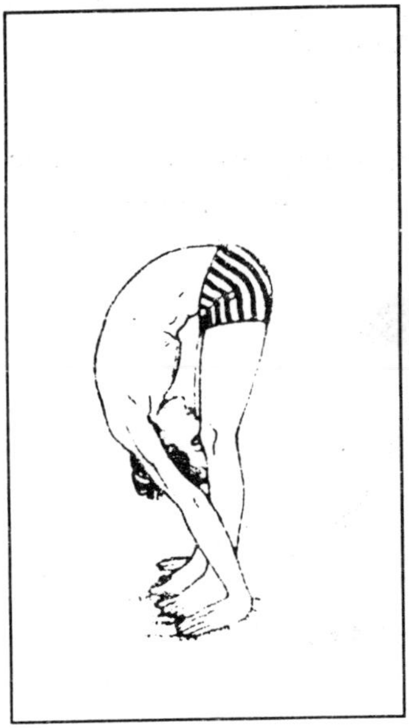

Fig. 16: Position 3

Position 4

Inhale and bend the left leg while stretching the right leg backwards with your toes and knees touching the ground. Lift your gaze towards the sky, bringing your awareness on the forehead centre. Do not release your breath.

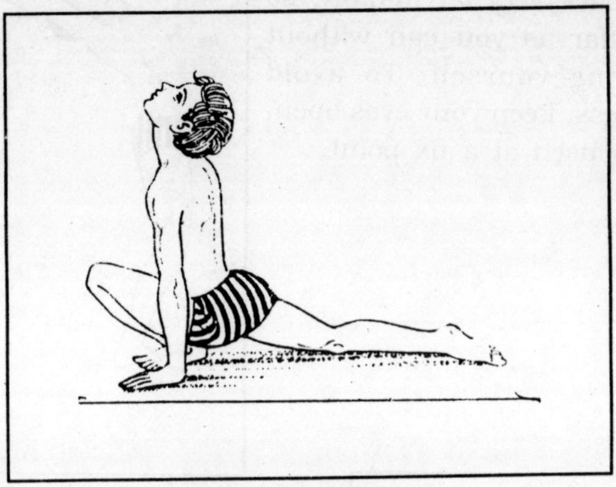

Fig. 17: Position 4

Position 5

Retain the breath. Move the other leg back, and lift

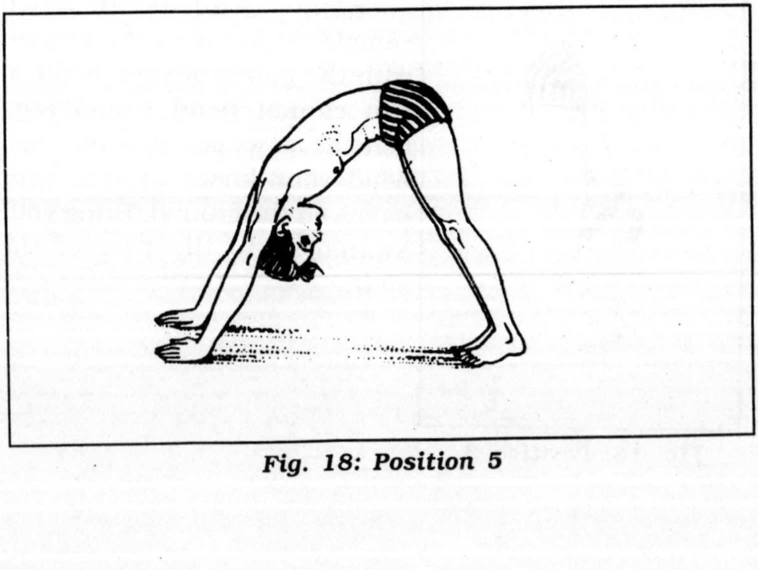

Fig. 18: Position 5

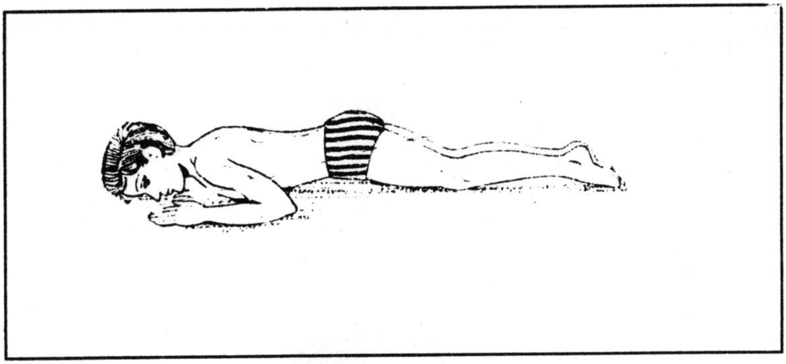

Fig. 19: Position 5

both the knees off the ground. The heels, hips, head move in one line, in a push-up position. Bring your awareness to the neck centre.

Position 6

Exhale and bring your body to the ground. In this position, known as Ashtanga namaskar, or eight curved positions. In this only eight part of the body touch ground—two feet, two knees, two hands, chest and forehead. In this the abdominal region is raised and, if possible, the nose is also kept off the ground, with only the forehead touching it. Bring your awareness to the navel.

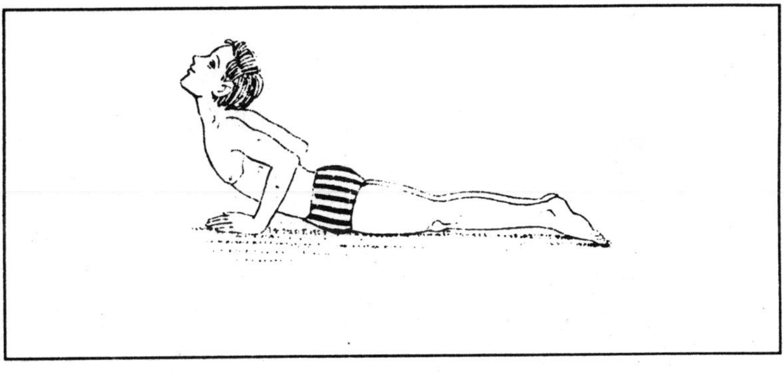

Fig. 20: Position 6

Position 7

Inhale while slowly raising your trunk, straighten the

arms and bend your head backwards. Bring your awareness to the root of the spine.

Position 8

Exhale and form an inverted 'V', as done in step 5, bring your awareness to the neck centre.

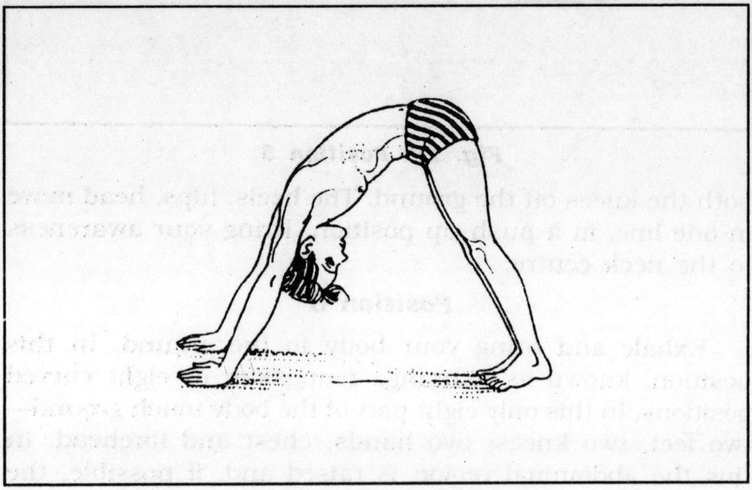

Fig. 21: Position 8

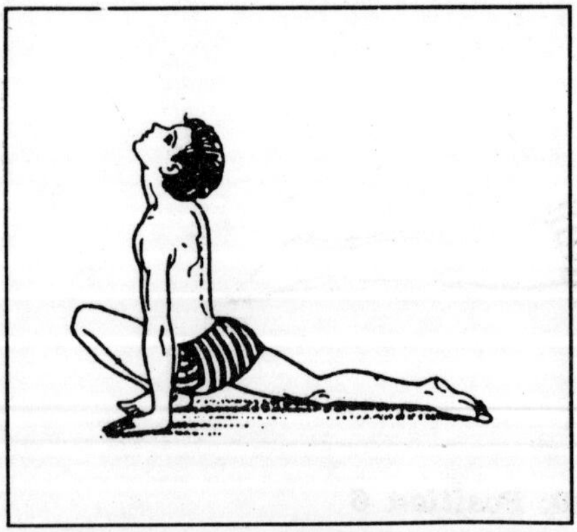

Fig. 22: Position 9

Position 9

Inhale and come down into the posture at step 4, folding the left leg and stretching the right leg. Bring your awareness to the forehead.

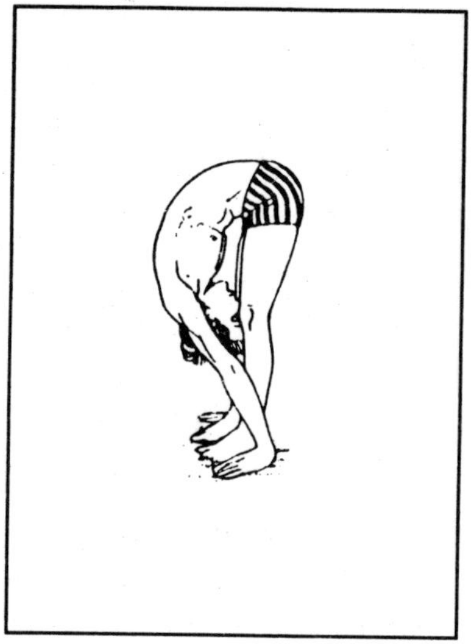

Position 10

Exhale and raise your body into the bending position as in step 3, bringing your awareness to the root of spinal column.

Fig. 23: Position 10

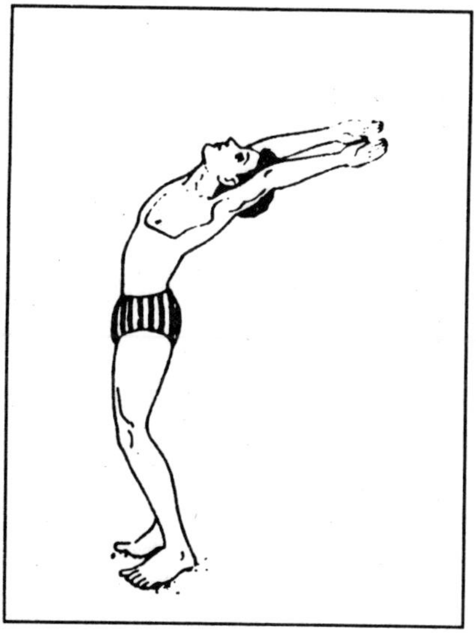

Position 11

Inhale and raise yourself completely stre-tching backwards as in step 2, and bring your awareness to the neck centre.

Fig. 24: Position 11

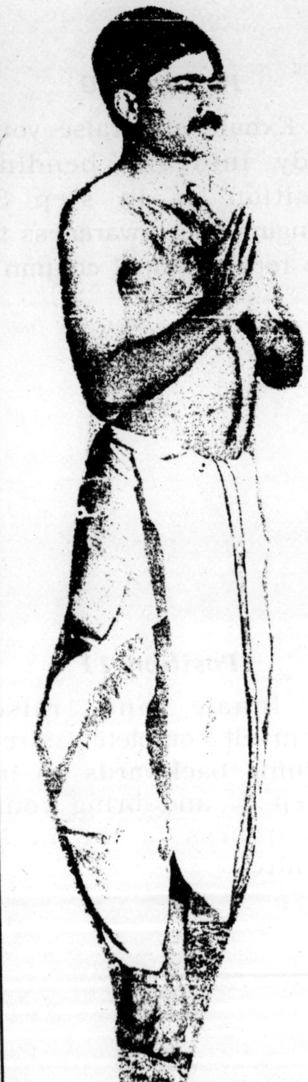

Position 12

Exhale and bring your hands in the same position as in step 1, bringing your awareness to the heart centre.

Fig. 25: Position 12

Dakshaasna

Bring your hands down to the side after each round of *Suryanamaskar*. Relax and visualize your body with your eyes closed. Begin the next round only after you feel prepared. Note that the position of hand on the ground remains at the same spot throughout one round. Start with 3 to 6 *Suryanamaskar* in a session, gradually increase the number of reptitions as the stamina builds up

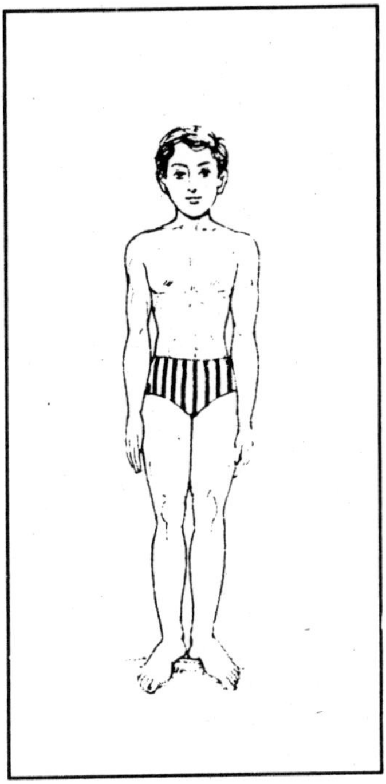

Fig. 26: Dakshaasna

CHAPTER 5

Hydrotherapy

The Nature Cure system of healing makes use of several remedial procedures external to the body. These procedures are designed to achieve two aims:

* Speed the process of healing and
* Providing relief to the patient from the painful symptoms of the disorder.

Among these external remedies prescribed by Nature Cure, hydrotherapy is of special importance. Water is a vital necessity of our life and health.

Nature cure provides various widely accepted methods of hydrotherapeutic treatment, most important among which are enema, hip-bath, the full sheet pack, local wet packs, steam-bath, hot foot bath, spinal bath, localised fomentation by steam, *jalaneti*, irrigation of the stomach, sponge bath, etc.

Before going into detail, let us consider the two common uses of water. These are: (1) drinking, and (2) bathing.

We must drink at least one and a half litre of water in a day. Best results are obtained if water is taken on an empty stomach just after getting up and cleaning the teeth, half an hour before each meal, and two hours after each meal. If you must drink water during the meals, then the quantity does not exceed 200 to 250 ml. In addition, of course, water can be taken as required when needed. The temperature of the water should preferably be neither too high nor too low. A glass of water with a little lemon juice, taken early in the morning on an empty stomach, is highly beneficial. Magnetised water would be even better. The method of magnetising water is given in detail in Chapter 15. No more than a mouthful or two of water may be taken during a meal if absolutely necessary. No water should be taken for one and a half to two hours after a meal, because it hampers digestion process.

Keep it in your mind that drinking water in quantities smaller than those indicated above leads to constipation, and has an adverse effect on the functioning of the kidneys.

Hip Bath

Hip-baths are very useful in stimulating the liver, spleen, intestines, kidneys, stomach and other digestive organs, and in maintaining their efficiency.

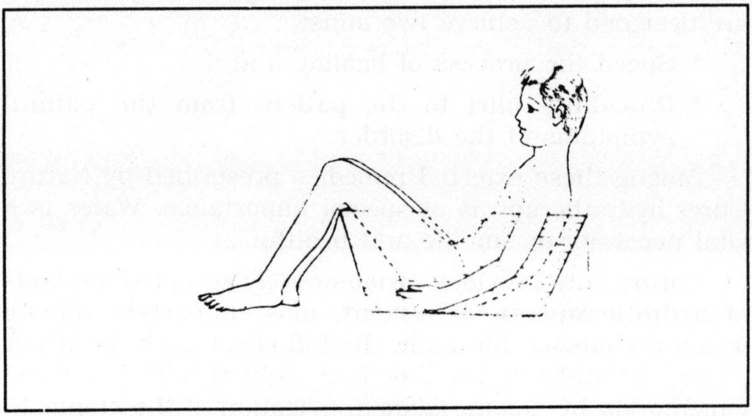

Fig. 27: Hip Bath

A special type of tub is required for a hip bath, the tub is oval in shape and one end of it is raised so that the bather can rest his back against it. If that is not available, the oval tubs used for collecting the used plates in parties etc. also serve satisfactorily. Normally the tub for a hip bath should be about 30 inches (75 cms) long and 20-22 inches (50cms) wide. The tub of above mentioned measurement is ideal for taking hip-bath.

Method

The tub should be filled with lukewarm water to a depth of 8-10 inches (20-25 cms). Drink a glass of warm water, and sit in the tub with the abdomen and part of the thighs submerged in the water, and the upper trunk and the legs outside the tub. Keep massaging the abdomen with some pressure, using a thick coarse towel or napkin.

* Nothing should be consumed for half an hour after a hip bath.

* Hot water hip-baths are very effective in abdominal pains, menstrual disorders or premature menopause, etc. While taking a hot water hip bath, a napkin wetted with cold water should be placed on the scalp. Alternate cold and hot hip-baths may prove beneficial in the disorders mentioned. Two tubs should be placed side by side for this purpose, and two minutes should be spent in each tub alternately.

* The stomach should always be empty while taking hip-bath.

* Take hip bath for ten to fifteen minutes in winter, and 20 to 30 minutes in summer. Dry yourself thoroughly after a hip-bath; a few exercises meant for toning up the abdominal organs may be undertaken.

Hot Foot Bath

This is an effective method of reducing congestion of blood or water in the upper parts of the body.

The water should be fairly hot, it should not be hot enough to cause pain or serious discomfort. Hot water sufficient to fill about three quarters of a large bucket, a woollen blanket and a napkin are the other requirements for hot foot bath.

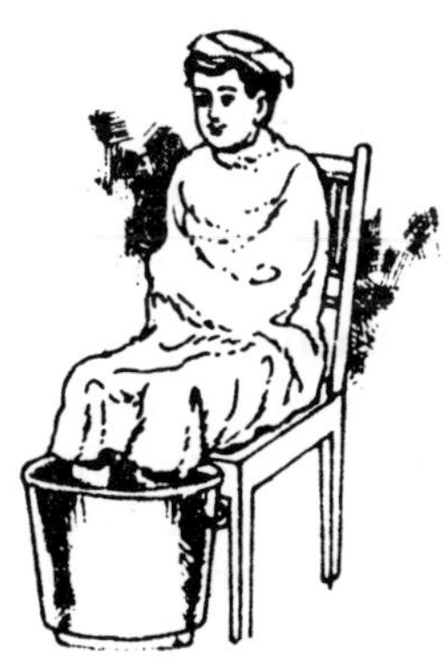

Fig. 28: Hot Foot Bath

Method

Put the bucket of hot water in front of a chair.

Drink a glass of warm water and sit on the chair with minimum clothing. Immerse both feet in the hot water. Wrap the blanket around the body and place a napkin wrung out in cold water on the scalp. If it is not possible to immerse both the feet in water at the same time, immerse them alternately one at a time. After a time, it should be possible to immerse both of them. In 15 to 20 minutes you will start perspiring. When a fair amount of perspiration has been formed, the bath can be terminated. Cold water should be sprinkled from time to time on the napkin placed on the head. Ladies should normally keep the hair dry (unoiled) while taking the hot foot bath. Alter the bath, the body must be wiped with a cold wet cloth, and one should lie down on bed for 5 to 10 minutes to relax.

* In case of insufficient perspiration in the expected time, take the feet out of the bucket, and pour 3 to 4 glasses of boiling water into the bucket. The higher temperature of water will do the job.

* The blood pressure goes down during the course of the bath. A feeling of giddiness therefore may ensue. This feeling will pass away on resting for a few minutes. But as a precautionary measure, very weak persons, pregnant women and patients with abnormal blood pressure should not take hot foot baths.

* Hot foot bath causes plenty of blood to rush to the feet. So there is no reason to worry if the feet remain red for 10 to 15 minutes after the hot foot bath.

Spinal Bath

The spinal column is a control centre for various messages to and from the body. The spinal bath strengthens, stimulates and nourishes the spine, thus indirectly benefiting the whole nervous system and the whole body.

A spinal bath tub, a bath towel and a blanket are required for spinal bath.

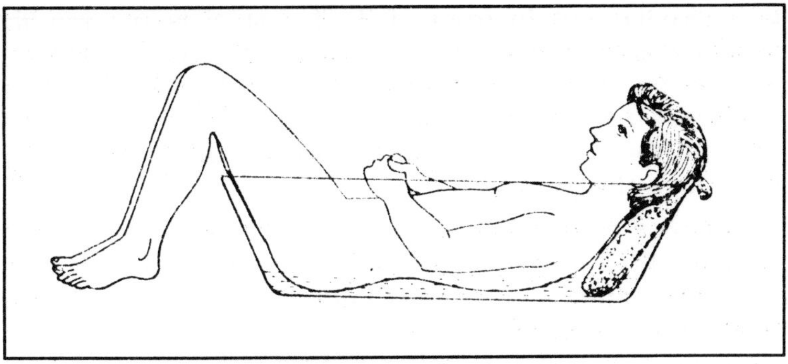

Fig. 29: The Spinal Bath

Method

The tub specially designed for the spinal bath is available in the market. The tub is wider at the top than at the bottom. Fill the tub to a depth of about two inches (5 cms). Lie down in the tub with the arms and the legs outside the tub. In this position, the entire spinal column with the exception of two or three vertebrae of the neck will be under the water level. Wet the bath towel, fold it lengthwise, and place it as a support for the neck and the head on the slanting wall of the tub. When the head is allowed to rest on the towel, the whole spine will immerse in the water. After taking up this position, cover the whole body except the head with a blanket, to protect the body from the outside draughts. The bath should last for about 10 to 15 minutes in winter, and 15 to 20 minutes in summer. During a spinal bath a pair of shorts can be worn.

In case of unavailability of a suitable tub, a spinal bath can still be taken, on the floor. A towel is wetted in cold water and folded lengthwise to form a 6 to 7 inch (15 cms) wide band. Spread this band on the floor and lie down on it in such a way that the towel is in contact with entire spine. The towel can be folded to a greater thickness under the neck. Then the body should be covered with a blanket as mentioned earlier.

Genitals Bath

Place a stool one foot long, six inches wide and six inches high in the tub. It would be much better if there is a circular cut in front of it. If a stool is not readily available keep four bricks, two upon two to raise the level and sit on them. The water level in the tub should be such that it is one inch above the stool. The water should be cold; the cool water from an earthen pitcher can very well serve the purpose.

Remove your clothes and sit on the stool. Take a piece of cloth, dip it in water and gently rub your abdomen with it for two minutes. Then take hold of the foreskin of your penis in two fingers and rub it lightly with a soft piece of cloth dipping cold water often. This can be continued for ten to twenty minutes. A lean person can do it for only ten minutes, and the hefty one for as long as twenty minutes. After the rubbing of the foreskin is completed, rub the entire spine with a wet towel for two minutes. You can take hold of the wet towel in two hands and move it up and down on your spine.

The ladies should rub their abdomen. They should take a piece of soft cloth, pull up the lips of the vagina and rub them slowly. And in the end they should also rub the spine as above. Hip bath or genitals bath should be avoided at the time of menstruation.

One must undertake exercise, walk or lie down on a bed and wrap himself in a blanket to restore the body heat lost due to immersion in water.

In case of unavailability of a tub, this bath can be taken in the sun. In that case spread a wet towel on the stool on which you sit. Keep a bucket full of water near the stool and take the bath as mentioned above.

Steam Bath

This is another widely accepted and useful method for the elimination of poisons from the body by inducing profuse perspiration. A specially designed cabinet or steam box is necessary for the steam bath. It can be purchased from the market, or can even be built at home.

Method

The patient must drink a glass of warm water and sit down in the cabinet with minimum or no clothing. A small towel wetted with cold water must be wrapped around the head to keep it cool. Cold water should be sprinkled from time to time on the head during the steam-bath. Now steam from the kettle should be let into the cabinet. When sufficient perspiration has been formed, which would be in about fifteen minutes or so, the bath should be discontinued. Excess should be avoided. After emerging from the bath, the body should be wiped with a wet cloth, or a cold bath should be taken. The body feels light and full of vigour after a steam bath. But remember that this bath should be taken when the stomach is empty.

* Though a steam bath is advisable once a week only, but fat persons may take it twice a week with advantage.

* Pregnant women, weak patients and patients suffering from heart ailments or from abnormally high or low blood pressure should avoid steam baths.

* In case of giddiness experienced during a steam bath, the bath should be terminated at once. The head should be washed with cold water and bed rest taken for some time, till one feels better.

* To eliminate of poisons from the body, the full sheet pack is considered to be of greater utility than the steam bath.

* Steam bath is an infallible method of increasing the metabolic rate and reducing weight.

* Use of a steam bath to bring down the temperature in fevers is totally unjustified.

How to Take a Bath

Bathing has quite an importance in our daily life. A bath is a daily ritual, but few people understand its purpose or importance. That is why most of us merely throw water over our heads and the bodies and think that we have done our duty.

The main purposes of a bath are: cleanliness and reactivating the circulation of the blood by the tingling sensation that cold water produces as it comes into contact with the skin. The first purpose, i.e., cleanliness, can be better served by hot water. The skin of the body has millions of pores through which the skin breathes as we do through our lungs. If the pores are clogged, the lungs are overworked. Overwork may lead to fatigue or exhaustion of the lungs. And then, closed pores do not pass any perspiration which is essential to clear the blood of morbid humours. Closed pores are a danger to the general health of human beings. Bathing also imparts a blissful feeling of freshness.

Frequent baths, with a good scrubbing during baths will keep the skin clean and glowing. Cold water is also a cleansing agent, but it cannot deal with the grease and dirt infesting the pores of the skin. Hot water mixed with lemon juice is the best cleansing agent for the skin. It would be better if you take a lemon and roast it lightly over a fire. Then cut it into two parts, dip a part in hot water and rub it over your skin. This will cleanse your skin as no soap can do. But a hot bath should not be taken daily. It generally brings lethargy, weakness and slows down the digestive processes. Once or twice a week is enough if you have to take a hot bath. The temperature of the water should not be more than one or two degrees above body temperature. A sparse use of soap is recommended. Multani clay, turmeric powder and cream may be used occasionally.

A hot bath before going to bed in the night is the best for health. It helps one to sleep better and if he covers his body after a hot bath, it will save him from the danger of exposure. A bath, hot or cold, should be taken one hour before meals or three hours after it.

Extremely hot water for a bath has its own advantages but it should be used sparingly. If one is suffering from a cold, he should take a hot bath, cover himself with woollens and get into bed. It will drive away the cold. A really hot bath when one is tired, drive away the fatigue.

A daily bath should be with cold water. When the skin is cooled by the cold water, blood rushes to warm it up. The circulation of the blood is activated and the blood is also cleansed of many impurities. A slowed down circulation is a prelude to old age. A cold bath is, therefore, instrumental in keeping one young.

Before having a bath rub the whole of body with palms or with a rough towel. Start with your scalp, forehead, face and the neck. Then go on to your wrists and then to the shoulders through the arms. Afterwards rub your chest, the armpits and abdomen and the back. The feet should be the last to receive attention. Keep your feet straight when you rub them. Start from the feet and come up to the thighs. In the beginning, rub gently but increase the pressure gradually.

After rubbing vigorously take a cold bath. Wipe your body with a towel. Start with the head and then dry up the whole body. You will feel a unique kind of pleasure when you rub your body after a bath. For weak persons a rubbing will be as good as exercise.

If right method of taking a bath is adopted, there will not be any danger of any skin eruptions or itch. The face will be free of pimples and other blemishes. The skin will acquire a healthy glow.

If you would use the palms of the hand to dry up the body after a bath instead of a towel, it will be extremely beneficial.

Enema

Constipation paves the way for many major and minor ailments. There is no other way to relieve constipation, and to get rid of the wastes that have accreted in the large intestine, which is as simple, as harmless, as effective and prompt, as the enema. It is difficult to predict exactly when a purgative will take effect; and it is easy to imagine the awkward situations that may arise when the effect manifests itself in unforeseen circumstances at the wrong time and in the wrong place. Moreover, if you do not take enema, you can derive no benefit from fasting or living on fruit diet alone.

An inexpensive apparatus for taking enemas is available in the market. It consists of an enamelled container for water (the fountain syringe, or the enema can), a plastic tube about 5 feet (1½ metres) in length, a tap for regulating the flow of water, and a catheter, or nozzle. A small bakellite catheter is available, but it would be more advisable to purchase a No. 24 plastic catheter, which is much more convenient.

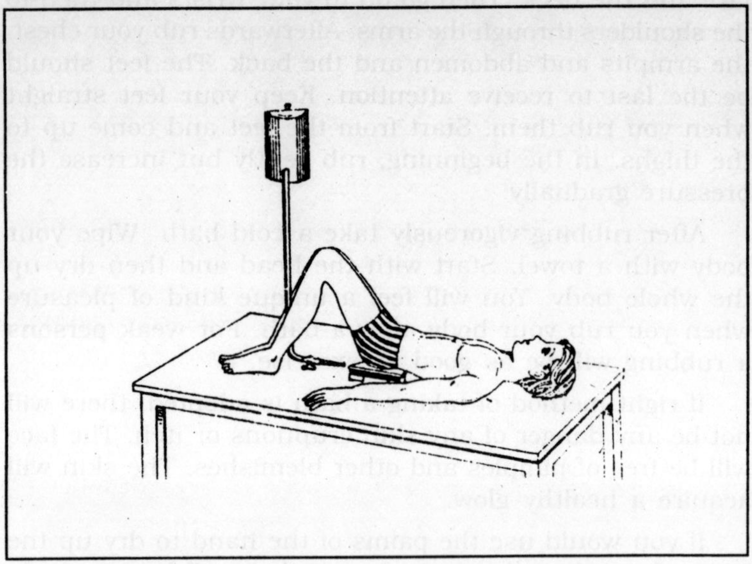

Fig. 30: Method of Taking an Enema

Method

Fill a litre and a half or two litres of lukewarm water in the container, and hang it at a height of about 3 feet (1 metre) from the floor, or place it on something of the required height. The end of the catheter should be lubricated with soap or oil. The anus should be similarly lubricated. Let some water escape from the catheter by opening the tap, so as to remove air bubbles if there any in the container.

Lie down flat on the floor or something hard as shown in the figure, with the hips slightly higher on a suitable support. Insert 3 to 4 inches (10 cm) of the catheter gently and carefully into the rectum. Open the tap. The water from the container will begin to flow into the large intestine. When all the water has been introduced, remove the catheter. Control yourself for two to three minutes even if you feel the urgency of elimination, and then visit the lavatory. All the water will be expelled, taking the wastes with it. Do not exert yourself at all to effect the ejection. Sit for a few minutes even after the outflow.

* A daily enema is essential two or three days prior to, and after the commencement of, a period of fasting or liquid diet regime. In acute diseases, enemas should be taken daily for 2-3 days. In chronic diseases, daily enemas may be necessary for a week or longer period.

* In comparison to purgatives enema is much more effective and harmless. There are no side effects. The results obtained in 10-11 minutes will be beyond expectation.

* Persons who take sufficient quantities of fibrous foods like fruits, vegetables, etc., or those who exercise regularly, in rare cases need enema.

* If there is requirement of enemas for a number of days, occasional addition of lemon juice to the water for the enema will help the thorough cleaning of the intestines. Except for lemon juice, nothing such as soap or similar things should ever be added to the water. The soda in the soap is harmful for intestines.

* Except exceptional circumstances, hot water enemas are not recommended.

Jalaneti

This procedure is extremely effective and beneficial for clearing of the upper parts of the respiratory system, viz., the nose and the throat.

A glass of lukewarm salt water and a small bowl are required for this procedure.

Method

A bowl should be filled to the brim with salt water. Dip the nose into the water, and immediately, without losing any time, draw up as much water as possible through the nose. Open the mouth immediately, and let the water that has been taken in flow out through the mouth. Keep doing the same till the glassful of water is used up. At the end, try to eject the water remaining in the nasal passages by blowing the nose.

Initially a feeling of suffocation is likely to be experienced for the first two or three days. The head may feel heavy and congested. But these discomforts will disappear in two or three days as one becomes habitual.

Sometimes a gradual increase in the amount of water is recommended by the experts. The aim should be to use up half a litre to a litre of salt water in this way. This usually proves beneficial.

One can perform *Jalaneti* at any time of the day. However, the early morning is the most suitable time for it. If the nose gets blocked up due to cold or any other reason, causing a difficulty in breathing, performance of *neti* at the time of going to bed would be preferable. Once you are accustomed to *Jalaneti*, if there is no other factor contra-indicating the change, it is permissible to use cold water in place of warm water occasionally for this purpose.

Some experts recommend that the water drawn in through the nose should be swallowed. But this is not advisable. In order to prevent the dirt collected in the nose from entering the digestive tract it is better to let the water out through the mouth.

Benefits

This procedure cleans the nose thoroughly. It is an effective remedy for colds. It relieves headache. It has a salutary effect on the eyes and sharpens vision. Congestion of the nose, other sundry ailments of the nose are other conditions which can be relieved by *Jalaneti*.

Irrigation of Stomach

About four glasses of warm water containing two teaspoonfuls of salt is required for this purpose.

Method

The most suitable time for this procedure is early morning, but it can be carried out at any other time provided the stomach is empty. Start gulping the salt water mentioned above, without interruption, making every effort to swallow as much of it as you possibly can, forcing the water down your throat, if necessary. It is essential that the water should be ingested continuously, not sip by sip. A stage will be reached when you find it absolutely impossible to take in even one more mouthful of water. You will also experience a feeling of nausea.

Bend down, and put the two middle fingers deep down your throat. This will at once cause the water to be vomited out. After all the water seems to have come out, try once or twice to induce vomiting again. Most of the water will be regurgitated by this method. The rest of it will be eliminated through the kidneys.

This procedure must be applied once or twice a month. In certain diseases many physicians recommend that the irrigation be carried out daily or on alternate days. This, however, is not desirable, because elimination of the residual salt water puts a great strain on the kidneys, and it may prove to be harmful.

Benefits

Many physicians believe that disturbances of digestion, and especially disturbances of the functions of the stomach, are at the root of all disorders. Vomiting clears the aesophagus and the stomach. It relieves asthma, acidity, dyspeptic belching, and many other ailments. Occasional irrigation of the stomach takes care of such complications.

Inhalation of Salt Water Steam

About four glasses of salt-water in a large vessel a large blanket and wet cloth for wiping perspiration are requires for this procedure.

Method

Put the salt water vessel on a stove. When the water comes to a boil place the vessel on the floor and sit down beside it. You should be wearing the minimum possible clothing. Cover your body and the vessel with a blanket like a tent. Keep your eyes closed and inhale the steam deeply. Lean over the vessel so as to let the vapour warm your face, the inside of the mouth, the nasal passages, and even the chest. There will be profuse perspiration in 5 to 7 minutes. Afterwords wipe the parts that have been exposed to the steam with a piece of cloth wrung in cold water.

Benefits

This is an effective remedy for cold. It is also useful in all types of disorders of the respiratory system. The fomentation caused by the steam is useful in curing pimples on the face, and relieves cough and asthma. Relief from toothache is also its main feature.

A Word of Caution

The persons who are suffering from hypertension or tuberculosis must not take the treatment for more than two or three minutes. Also, they should inhale the steam through the mouth and the nose, but should never expose the chest to the vapours.

Wet and Dry Fomentation with Hot Water

This method is very useful for relief of localised pain or for improving the circulation in a part of the body where for some reason the circulation has become sluggish. Covering the painful region with cloth dipped in hot water, subjecting the region to the action of steam from a special kettle, or applying heat by means of a hot-water bag or bottle results in sedation of the muscles, improvement in circulation and reduction of swelling. As a consequence, pain is relieved. After the fomentation, the part subjected to the treatment must be wiped with a cloth soaked in cold water.

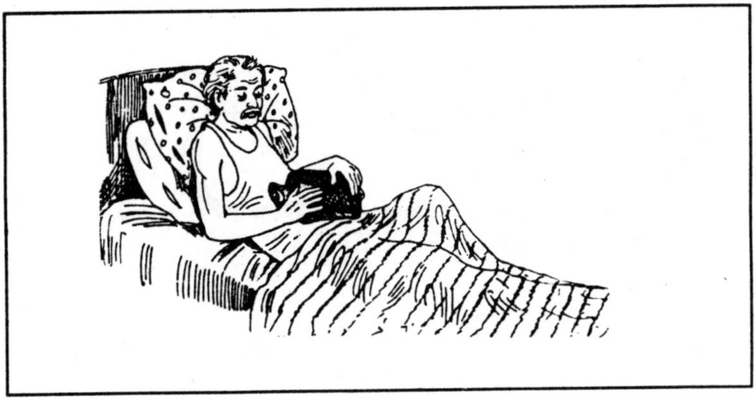

Fig. 31: Hot Fomentation

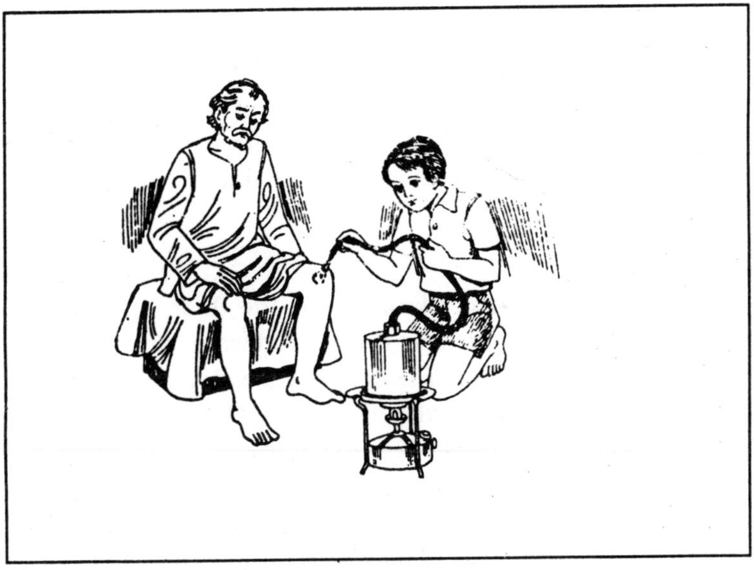

Fig. 32: Fomentation with Steam

Full Sheet Pack

Full sheet pack is a very effective means of eliminating the toxins in the body through perspiration.

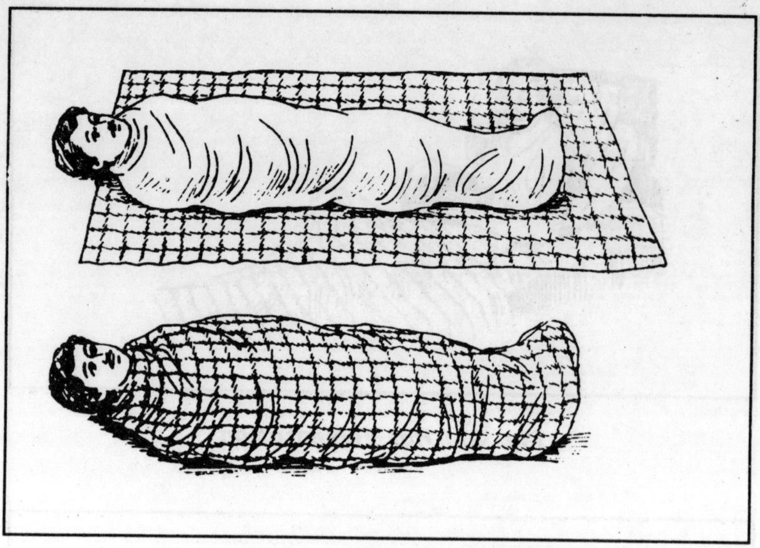

Fig. 33: Full Sheet Pack

The requirements are, a cotton sheet about 7 to 8 feet long and about four feet wide (2½ metres × 1¼ metres), one or two woollen blankets, and a napkin for the full sheet wet pack.

Method

After spreading the blankets on the floor, spread the sheet over them after wetting it with cold water and wringing it. Drink a glass of warm water, and lie down face up on the sheet in the nude, with the arms along the sides of the body. The head should lie outside the sheet get someone to wrap the sheet tightly around the body. The blankets must then be wrapped similarly around the body. The napkin should be wrung in cold water and wrapped around the scalp.

One may feel cold for a short time when wrapped up in this way, but soon the pack will begin to be warmed by the body heat. In 15 to 20 minutes he will begin to perspire freely. The perspiration will be soaked up by the sheet. The pack should be removed after 25 to 30 minutes and the body wiped with a piece of wet cloth. Large amounts of poisons in the body are eliminated through the perspiration.

Some Suggestions

* The cloth used for the pack must be washed thoroughly, and dried, before future use.

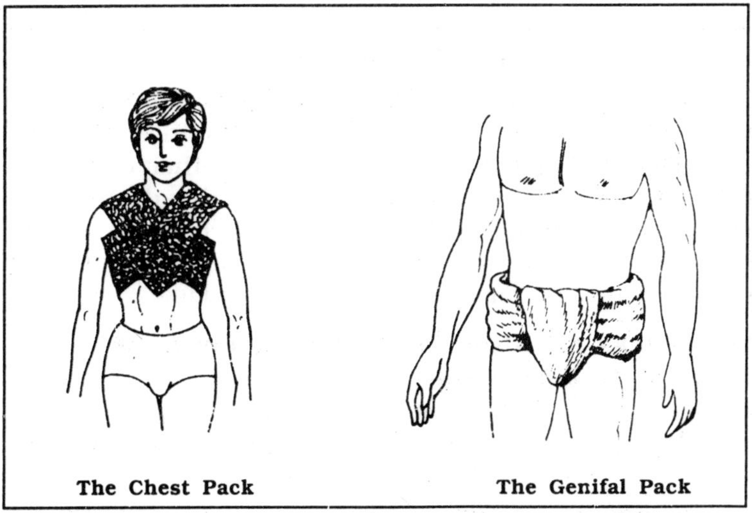

Fig. 34

* Local wet packs for the chest, abdomen, genitals or the arms and legs may be applied if necessary. The genital wet pack is also called the 'T Pack'.

* The main effect of the full sheet pack is the elimination of the toxic substances in the body through perspiration. If there is a fever, the pack will bring the temperature down by eliminating the poisons. But the pack should not be employed in the initial stages of the fever when the patient is shivering or feeling chill.

Clay Therapy

Clay or mud is as important as water as an external healing agent. The benefits derived from clay therapy are very much like hydrotherapy.

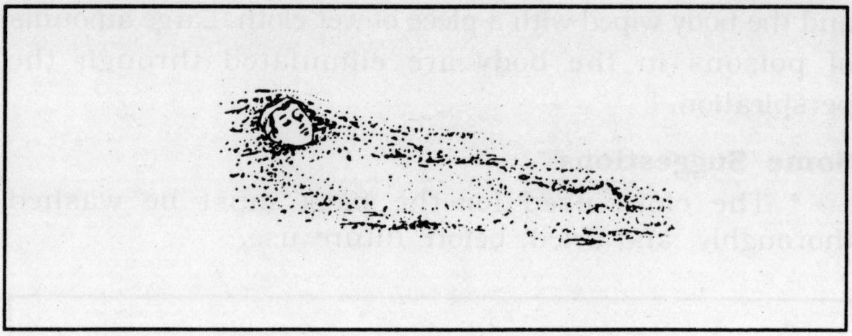

Fig. 35: Clay Therapy

In the form of paste, clay can be applied directly as a salve, or in the form of a pack, or as poultice. Usually, clay paste is applied to the abdomen or other regions of the body which exhibit symptoms of the disorder. If necessary, it can be applied to the whole body, or a mud bath can be taken, in which the entire body except head is buried in clay for treatment or relaxation.

Mud Packs are Used for Following Purposes

To Reduce Swelling: Clay pack is capable of reducing the swelling of any part of the body. This property of clay is well worth trying out by application of clay packs to swollen feet, or other parts of the body.

For Absorbing Toxins: Clay has the unique quality of absorbing toxins from the body. Proof of this power of clay is afforded by the fact that if clay is applied to a boil or a suppurating wound, the pus is quickly drawn out and the wound gets clean.

To Cool Affected Part: The mud pack has greater cooling effects than a wet pack. In case of high fever, the temperature can be brought down with the help of a mud pack. Of course, the mud pack will have to be changed frequently till the desired lowering of temperature has taken place.

Relieves Pain: Use of clay paste or a mud pack gives immediate relief from localised pain.

Relaxation: A clay pack effectively reduces the tension of the muscles and soothes overstimulated nerves.

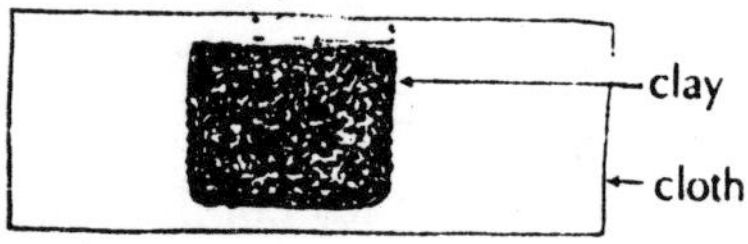

Fig. 36: The Clay Pack

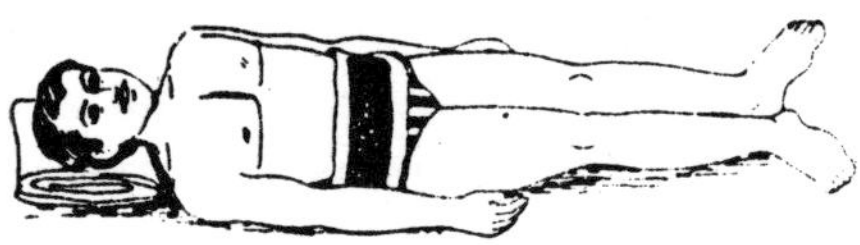

Fig. 37: Abdominal Clay Pack

The best way to prepare mud pack is to take clay from about four inches below the surface of the earth. Clay of any colour can be used for this purpose, provided it does not contain harmful materials or chemicals like compost, pebbles, etc. If the clay is highly viscous, some fine sand should be mixed with it.The clay should be sieved so as to remove pebbles, stones and other coarse materials from it. It should then be dried in the sun. When preparing the clay for application as a paste or pack, just enough water should be added to it to give it the consistency like soft dough. Then it should be spread over the affected part, to a thickness of about an inch (2.5 cms). Or it can be spread on a piece of fine cloth like muslin. If clay is to be applied over the eyes, the cloth is necessary.

If you would leave clay paste or pack is uncovered, it has a cooling effect on the affected part. But if it is covered well with thick cotton or woollen cloth, generally a warming effect is developed. If, therefore, the aim is to cool the part or reduce the temperature of the body, the clay should be left uncovered. But if a warming effect is desired, it should be covered. Normally, the clay should be used for 20 to 30 minutes or one hour. Clay can be applied afresh also if it is necessary.

If clay has been used for its cooling effect, the part to which it has been applied should first be wiped clean with a piece of cloth, and then brought to normal temperature by a dry rubbing with the palms. If it has been used for warming the part, the part should be wiped clean with cloth soaked in cold water and wrung afterwards.

Clay therapy has been found quite effective in constipation, diarrhoea, gastric, duodenal and intestinal ulcers, bleeding of the uterus, piles, fissures, appendicitis, stomachache, fevers, irregularity in menstruation and such other disorders. The beneficial effects of the use of clay on boils, wounds, pain or swellings have been found up to the mark. Clay is found in different colours in different places, but no matter whatever the colour, it is quite beneficial.

Massage

Another important remedial procedure in nature cure is massage. Massage has been used therapeutically for thousands of years all around the world.

The Effect of Massage on Organs and Systems of the Body

The Heart: Massage reduces the burden on the heart, and it is able to increase its efficiency to a great extent.

The Digestive System: Abdomen massage stimulates the digestive system, and promotes better elimination of wastes. The resistive powers of the body are strengthened due to the increase in the working capacity of the liver.

Skin: The beneficial effects of massage on the skin are widely known. The pores of the skin are opened up, it is good for the elimination of poisons from the body through sweat.

Muscles: With a massage the tension in the muscles can be reduced and one can be relieved of muscular pain. Strenuous exertion results in the accumulation of lactic acid in the muscles. Massage helps to rid the muscles of this acid and thus imparts a feeling of freshness, vigour and lightness.

Circulation of the Blood: The blood circulation in the part being massaged can be accelerated, so that the part is supplied with more nutrients, and its healing powers are augmented. The accelerated circulation reduces swelling. There is an increase in the capacity of the blood to carry oxygen for effective use.

Nerves: Gentle and slow massage with light pressure relieves tension of the nerves and soothes them. Vigorous massage stimulates lax nerves and increases their efficiency to a great extent.

The Urinary System: Urinary system can be activated by massage. As a result the process of elimination of toxic substances from the body through the urine is accelerated by the formation of greater quantities of urine.

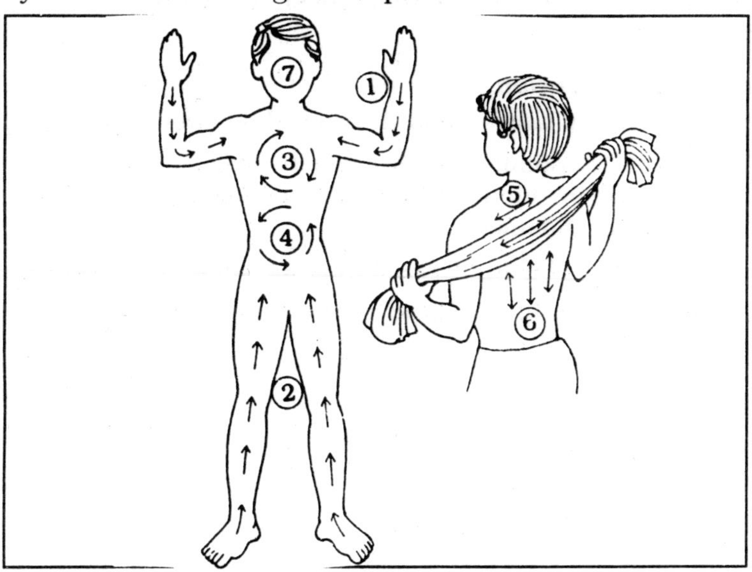

Fig. 36: Direction of movements in massage

Method

Start this process with massage of the arms and legs. Then the chest, abdomen, back and buttocks should be massaged, in that order, end with the face and the head. Cloth should be used for massaging the back. We should massage ourselves with our own hands to derive the benefits of massages as well as exercise.

Dry palms are okay for massage; but if the skin is too dry or if the body is excessively weak, wet cloth or soothing oil may be used. Among oils, sesame (til) oil is the best for this purpose. Some people use talcum powder for reducing friction while massaging, but this practice is not recommended, as the pores of the skin get clogged up with powder.

The appropriate directions of movements and sequence recommended for massaging the various parts of the body are shown in Fig. 36.

* After massage take a bath with lukewarm water.

If you are a patient of high blood pressure, then the direction of massaging movements should be reversed, i.e. from head to foot.

A Word of Caution

* Pregnant ladies should avoid abdominal massage.
* Avoid abdominal massages in cases of diarrhoea, gastric or duodenal ulcers, appendicitis or tumours in the abdomen.
* In cases of skin diseases massage should be avoided.

No massage of any kind is recommended in fevers.

CHAPTER 6

Air-Bath

Air is of prime importance for life. A man may survive without food for weeks, without water for days, but it is impossible to survive even for a minute or two without air.

Oxygen is necessary for the process of combustion taking place in all the various cells of the body. We obtain this oxygen from the air. When we inhale, oxygen of the air dissolves in the blood flowing through the fine capillaries in the lungs, and is thus carried to every cell in the body.

The ozone in the air helps the lungs to cleanse blood of carbon dioxide. Carbon dioxide and other toxic substances are formed in the cells as the end products of combustion and other processes taking place in the cells. Carbon dioxide thus formed dissolves in the blood. When this impure blood carrying carbon dioxide reaches the lungs, carbon dioxide is released into the air present in the lungs, and is expelled with it.

Hence, when we breathe in, oxygen of the air enters the lungs and dissolves in the blood. When we breathe out, carbon dioxide formed in the body is expelled. In brief, the blood gets purified in the lungs. Even this elementary information is sufficient to make you realize the importance of deep breathing.

On earth the main source of oxygen is vegetation such as trees, shrubs and other green plants. Plants take up carbon dioxide from the air for their nutrition and growth, and release oxygen into the air. The proportion of oxygen in the atmosphere is, hence, somewhat greater in areas having more greenery. Densely populated on the other hand, are comparatively deficient in oxygen, and polluted in other ways. The thoughtless and wanton destruction of vegetation going on today aggravates this deficiency and pollution.

A walk in open areas covered with greenery, such as gardens and fields, is highly beneficial, especially when accompanied by deep breathing to ventilate the lungs. The cool breeze of early mornings, being fresh, pure and rich in oxygen, purifies the blood and the body, and fills our minds with sense of well-being. The salubrious effects of fresh air on the body, mind and health are widely acknowledged.

Some Suggestions

* You should not cover the face while sleeping.

* Keep the windows open in winters.

* One should always take deep breaths. The breathing of most city people leading sedentary lives is shallow. The result is that carbon dioxide is not eliminated properly, and toxins consequently accumulate in the body to give birth to future problems.

* One should always breathe through the nose. The hair in the nose performs the function of a filter, removing the fine dust particles in the air. Moreover, the air gets warmed up in passing through the nasal passages, which has a salutary effect in the lungs.

CHAPTER 7

Sun-Bath

Sunlight is essential for revitalising human body. Sunlight gives the green colour to the plants and gives red to our blood. Sunlight is of great importance for perfect health. How useful and indeed essential, sunlight is in our life, finds no place in our thoughts. In consequence we invite diseases, generally by wilful neglect of this most healthful gift of nature bestowed freely upon us everywhere. Just as a plant withers away without it, a human being deprived of it will be pale, wan, and sickly.

The Type of Sun Rays

1. *Infra-red rays:* These rays impart heat. The warmth of these rays is soothing in the winter. Moreover, these rays relax and soothe the muscles, reduce swelling and give relief from pain.

2. *Rays of visible (white) light:* This light of the sun is made up of light of seven different colours, as seen in the rainbow. Every colour has its particular effect on the body.

3. *Ultra-violet rays:* These are of special importance. Vitamin D is produced in the body by the action of ultra-violet rays falling on the skin. Sunlight is the best source of Vitamin D. A deficiency of Vitamin D causes a disease of the bones known as 'Rickets'. Ultra-violet rays are necessary for the healthy condition of the skin. The people who tend to keep their bodies covered from head to foot suffer from variety of skin diseases.

Sunlight helps greatly in the proper formation of teeth, rapid growth of hair, and quick and deep breathing. By the action of sunlight, skin diseases are cured, blisters are burst and wounds are healed more quickly. Sunlight maintains and even increases the amount of alkali in the blood. Hence, sunlight is life-giving gift of nature.

People disregard the importance of sunlight. Some people avoid going out in the sun for fear of darkening the skin, or if they do, they carry umbrellas etc. One should not overdress so that sunlight can replenish his vital force.

If an expecting mother takes sun baths regularly, she gets relief from the usual discomforts of pregnancy such as fatigue, backache, nausea, overstimulation (or overexcitement), etc. and lactation in the post-parturition period is also improved to a great extent.

In nutshell, whether it is a question of the development of a child or convalescence after a disease has been brought under control, sunlight helps to nourish and strengthen the body. After sleep, sunlight is the element which helps restore our vital force.

The whole body derives benefits from sunlight. Exposure to sunlight improves health and augments the resistive powers of the body.

An expert says, "The incidence of cancer is lower in those regions of the world where there is abundant sunshine all the year round. Diseases readily enter the dwellings that sunlight does not. Rickets and tuberculosis take up permanent residence, the incidence of pneumonia increases, and the infant death-rate goes up, in dwellings where darkness reigns. Contagious diseases spread much more quickly in dark and narrow lanes."

Even common disorders turn into virtulent forms among people who are deprived of sunlight and have to spend most of their time in the dark. When sufficient sunlight is not available, the proportions of fibrin and red blood corpuscles in the blood decrease, and those of white blood corpuscles and water increase.

Some Suggestions

* Start sun-bathing by exposing the body to the sunlight for 5 to 10 minutes, the anterior parts of the body for half this period and the posterior parts for the other half. Later on, the period of exposure can be gradually increased, as convenient, for up to an hour.

* If you feel giddiness, fatigue or discomfort experienced during a sun-bath, or a burning sensation in the skin, then it is an indication of excessive exposure to sunlight, in such cases sun bath should be discontinued.

* Mild sunlight of the early morning or the evening has no harmful effect on the body. It is always beneficial. But avoid exposing the body to the intense sunlight of the noon.

* See to it that your head is covered and the eyes closed while taking a sun-bath. Do not cover the face, and avoid looking directly at the sun.

* Try to take sun-baths without any clothes on. But if that is not possible, then minimum possible clothes should be worn.

* Take a cold water bath after sun-bath or wipe the body with a piece of cloth wrung out in cold water.

Sunlight helps nourish the muscles. If you would regularly bask in the sun, it will help to develop the size and strength of the muscles, and increases the proportion of calcium in them, giving them greater endurance. If the skin is deprived of sunlight by keeping it covered, the muscles tend to weaken and degenerate. Hence, use this free gift of nature whenever it is possible to restore your vital force.

CHAPTER 8

Magnetotherapy

Today magnetotherapy has become a popular remedial procedure. The basic tenet of the system is that one remains healthy so long as an equilibrium is maintained in the electromagnetic forces flowing in the body. Illness results from a disturbance of this equilibrium.

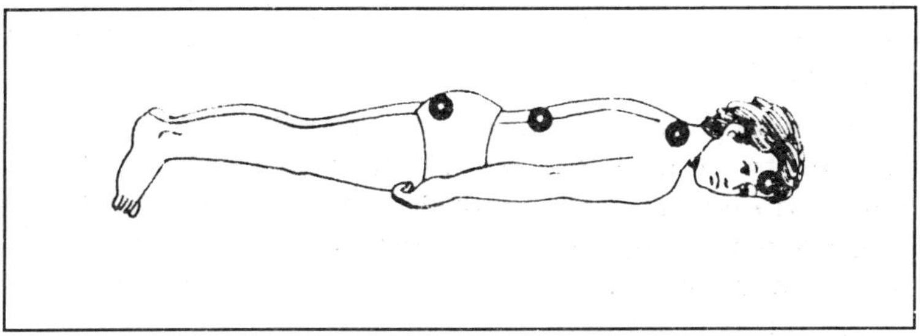

Fig. 39: Locations for Placing the Magnets

Magnets have been in use since age for the treatment of certain diseases. But scientific experiments to test the healing powers of magnets have been undertaken only in recent years. The discoveries of researchers filled them with joy.

Now it is an established fact that the electromagnetic waves emitted by magnets affect living organisms. Frequently there are magnetic storms on the surface of the sun. That these magnetic storms have profound effects on the animal life on the earth. Studies undertaken at institutes of India have established that during period of violent magnetic storms on the sun, the incidence of heart attacks increases. The unavoidable inference is that physical and mental disturbances on earth are associated with magnetic storms of the sun. The likelihood of perturbations of the heart, blood vessels, brain and nerves also increases to great extent. There had been numerous experiments to determine the effects of artificial magnets on plants, animals, and especially, humans. The region in the vicinity of a magnet is known as its 'magnetic field'. If seeds are kept for more than four hours in a 'magnetic field', they are found to grow more quickly. Precisely similar results are obtained if water that has been subjected to the action of magnets is used to water seeds after they are sown. If flies or mosquitoes are given food that has been 'magnetised' in this manner, they are found to live longer. Magnetic fields have beneficial effects on birds and animals too, birds becoming larger and stronger, cows yielding more milk, horses and bulls becoming more muscular and more powerful. Scientists have had notable success in arresting the growth of cancerous cells in animals, and in some cases even curing cancer, with the help of powerful magnets.

Many experiments have been carried out to ascertain the effects of magnets on human beings. It has been demonstrated by many controlled experiments that blood pressure is brought within the normal range, the proportion of red blood corpuscles is increased and that of cholesterol in the blood is reduced by systematic use of magnets.

How to Use Magnets

Physicians have developed various systems based on their own experiments and experiences for using magnets therapeutically.

It has been found by the experiments carried out so far that no matter what detailed procedure is adopted in using magnets therapeutically, there is a definite and undeniable effect on the entire body. An advantage of this therapy is no danger of any adverse side effects.

There are two therapeutic procedures: (1) the Unipolar method, using either one of the poles, and (2) the Bipolar

Method, using both the north and the south pole together, i.e. the method utilizing the whole magnetic field.

Before going into details about these two methods, it is necessary to know about the properties and effects of each pole.

Qualities of the South Pole

* The 'south pole' means 'stop'.
* It has a cooling and tranquillizing effect.
* The south pole possesses resistive and decelerating powers.
* It has a contractional effect.
* If this pole is put in ordinary water for a while, the alkalinity of water is increased. In other words, the south pole reduces acidity.
* Fruits, vegetables, etc. remain fresh for long periods if kept in the field of a south pole.
* It slows down the circulation of blood in the capillaries.
* It brings infection under control and reduces swelling.
* It controls and arrests the growth of tumours.

Qualities of the North Pole

Properties of north pole are generally opposite to those of the south pole.

* The 'north pole' means 'Go Ahead', 'Advance'.
* It gives warmth and energy and stimulates the physiological reactions.
* If the north pole is put in water for a while and the water tested with a pH indicator, it is found to be acidic. Thus, it has the effect of reducing alkalinity.
* It has the property of favouring expansion.
* It speeds up the circulation of blood in the capillaries.
* Fruits ripen quickly, vegetables begin to decay and milk begins to turn sour if kept in the magnetic field of north pole.

* It accelerates the growth of both benign and malignant tumours. The tumour, therefore, develops, and may possibly come to a head, burst and heal, or may even spread fast.
* It increases the possibility of infection, as it gives warmth and energy to germs also. It increases swelling.

The stimulating and warmth-giving effect of north pole proves useful in cases of hernia, leucoderma, allopasia, muscular dystrophy, paralysis general debility and debility following diseases, fainting, fits, etc.

In cases of infection and inflammatory conditions the south pole proves to be extremely useful. It is also beneficial in arthritis, infectious conditions, tumours, anxiety, convulsions, skin diseases, eye defects, eye diseases, insomnia, neuralgia, etc.

Many therapists have adopted the bipolar method of treatment. This method too has proved successful in curing certain disorders, though it takes more time to effect cures.

Most of the Indian magnetotherapists follow the unipolar method. According to them, the unipolar method may succeed in cases in which the bipolar method had been a failure.

The treatment of any specific disease or disorder, the use of a single pole is comparatively more logical. Before attempting any magnetotherapeutic procedure, it is absolutely necessary that the specific cause of the disorder be ascertained. If the unipolar method of treatment is to be adopted, a precise diagnosis becomes all the more necessary, as the use of the wrong pole may prove harmful for the patient.

If there is need of the bipolar method, i.e. to the utilisation of the entire magnetic field, then this method may be adopted without any misgiving. In cases where both pain and weakness or stiffness occur together, simultaneous treatment with both the poles is definitely advantageous, but there should not be any infection in the part being treated. The treatment will be more effective if the north pole faces the north and the south pole faces the south.

There is another procedure in magnetotherapy that is alternate treatment with the north and the south poles. This method, too, is recommended only when both pain and weakness or stiffness occur together, as indicated above. For treating injuries like cuts and contusions, and vertebral pain, backache, etc., the south pole can be applied for the first 15 to 20 minutes, and then the north pole for the same period. This alternation is similar to the alternate hot-and-cold bath treatment in hydrotherapy.

The particular method of using magnets for treatment depends on the particular disease and the symptoms described by the patient. It is also necessary that there should be regular examination of the patient by the therapist, and the method of treatment modified according to the changes noted in the symptoms of the disease.

The Seven Chakra in Body

Chakra	*Location*	*Magnetic pole*
Vishuddha	On the spine, at the base of the neck	Strong north pole
Manipura	On the spine, exactly behind the navel	Strong north pole
Swaadhish-thaana	Three inches above the lower end of the spine	Strong north pole
Aajnyaa	Midpoint of the forehead	Weak south pole

There are seven chakras in our body which regulate the electromagnetic forces and energies in the body. Daily stimulation of four of these chakras, viz., the *Vishuddha*, *Manipura*, *Swaadhishthaana* and *Aajnyaa* chakras, for about 15 to 20 minutes by magnets maintains the equilibrium of the electromagnetic forces in the body, thus assisting in the maintenance of health. See the table given above for details.

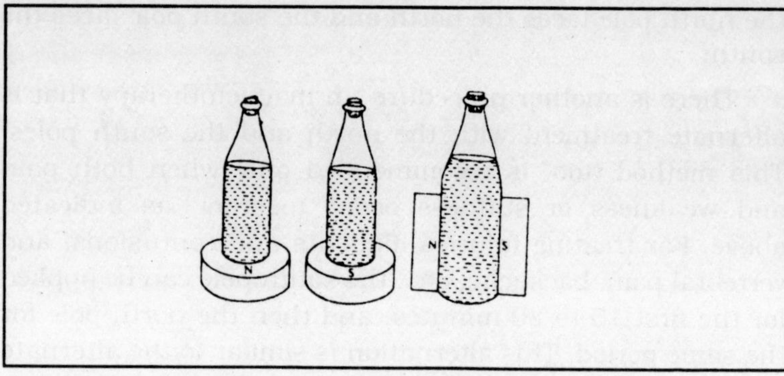

Fig. 40: Way of Magnetising Water

To 'Magnetise' the water for this purpose keep magnets in contact with the bottles or glasses filled with water for at least twelve hours. Besides drinking, this magnetised water can be used with advantage for cleaning the eyes, sprinkling on burns and washing wounds.

'Magnetised' water (i.e., water which has been subjected to the action of the north and the south poles), can also consumed three to four times a day to maintain good health. I hope that you will derive tremendous benefit by trying this simple method of maintaining health.

Venereal Diseases

Venereal diseases are the diseases which are communicated through sexual intercourse—those suffering from them are apt to hide them. It leads to their spreading on the one hand and the risk of their becoming chronic because of the desire of the patient to keep them secret. In India, little attention is paid to sex education, most people are ignorant of the functioning of the reproductive system beyond a hazy idea that the reproductive organs are a source of pleasure. Thousands of advertisements of remedies to deal with minor ailments like night emissions and phosphaturia. The ignorance of the common man on the subject of sex has proved highly beneficial to the unscrupulous and ignorant quacks. They scare people by telling them that night emissions and the presence of phosphates in the urine are dangerous. All systems of medicine except homoeopathy and naturopathy are geared to the suppression of the venereal disease through the use of harmful drugs which, besides killing the germs that are supposed to cause them, injure the system in devious ways. Nature cure can effectively deal with the venereal disease.

Gonorrhoea

Gonorrhoea and syphilis are two major diseases. Gonorrhoea is an inflammatory disease affecting specially the mucous membrane of the urethra in the male and that of the vagina in the female. But it spreads to other parts of the body also. It is a contagious disease transmitted by one person to another person, usually through sexual intercourse. It can also be passed on through the discharge on sponges, towels or clothing of the sufferer. In men it is characterised by irritation in the urethra, scalding pain on passing urine and a viscid discharge yellowish-white in colour. The glands in the groin often enlarge and may also suppurate. The urine is cloudy and threads of pus are visible to the naked eye. If the disease is not treated in the primary stage, various forms of inflammation in the neighbouring organs may appear, the testicles, prostate gland and the bladder becoming affected. At a later stage the inflammation of the urethra is liable to lead to gradual formation of fibrous tissue around the channel stopping the passeage altogether and making it impossible to urinate. Some of the joints of the body may become inflamed as the poison spreads into the system. Abscesses may appear on the body and the valves of the heart may become inflamed.

In females, it is characterised by a yellow discharge from the vagina, painful urination and inflammation of the glands situated close to the opening of the vagina. The inflammation may spread to the uterus, the fallopian tubes and the ovaries causing permanent destructive changes in these and leading occasionally to peritonitis—inflammation of the membrane covering the abdomen—through the fallopian tubes, which is a serious conditon.

Syphilis

Syphilis is another major disease, it is also equally contagious. At the time of commencement it shows a characteristic sore at the site of the infection. In advanced stages, it produces morbid conditions similar to those produced by leprosy and tuberculosis. The disease affects only human beings and is communicated, like gonorrhoea, through sexual intercourse with the affected person.

It may be acquired from persons already suffering from it or it may be inherited from one or both parents. It is acquired usually through sexual intercourse, though cases are not rare where it has been passed on through kissing or contact with the syphilitic sores of another person. Articles used by the person suffering from syphilis are also carriers of the disease for some period.

Initially a small ulcer appears at the site of the infection which is accompanied by a typical hardness of tissues immediately around and beneath it, and characterised by resistance to all healing treatment. This is the primary stage of syphilis. The sore may not occasion any discomfort and may even go unnoticed. But after some time, lymphatic glands round the sore and also all over the body become swollen and hard. This condition may last for some weeks, after which the secondary stage of the complication starts. It commences with fever and loss of appetite, vague pains throughout the body and a faint red rash seen best on the chest. From here onwards, the spread of the disease is quick; the hair may start falling and there may be bloodlessness, the appearance of sores in the mouth and the throat, headache and mental deterioration. There may also be painful swelling in the bones.

The final stage develops after the lapse of some months or years. Masses of granulation tissue appear throughout the body. They are hard nodules or there may be tumour-like masses in the muscles. The final blow, is the diseases of the nervous system and the arteries.

When the infection is transferred through heredity, the child might be a dead birth, or the woman may abort or have a miscarriage. If ever the child is born, a few weeks after its birth, the symptoms of second stage appear.

Treatment

In the old times sulphonamides and compounds of mercury and arsenic were used to deal with the venereal diseases. It was only during the Second World War when penicillin was tried in the treatment of these diseases with some success. Later a whole range of broad-spectrum antibiotics have been employed by physicians to deal with syphilis and gonorrhoea. In the indigenous system of medicine, many compounds of poisonous substances and oxides of various metals were tried, but no remarkable success had been achieved. The best that these remedies have been able to do is to act as palliatives, giving temporary relief. But what is worse, they have acted to suppress the diseases which later manifest themselves to pose more serious threat on sufferers life.

Start the treatment by reforming the mentality of the patient first. He must be persuaded to lead a clean life and abstain from sexual intercourse. He should also see to it that none of his personal articles—particularly items of apparel and towels—are used by others so that the infection does not spread to innocent persons of his family or people of his circle.

Initially these diseases appear as disorders of the skin and it is only later, when suppressive drugs have been administered to the patient, that they become chronic or affect other parts of the body. The next step in their treatment must, therefore, be the cleansing of the blood. That is possible only through proper regulation of the diet. Fruits and vegetables are the best agents for expelling the poisons from the blood stream. But heavy fruit-like, bananas, jackfruit, sugarcane and potatoes should be avoided in the beginning. Musk melon is the best fruit which should be the mainstay of the diet of a person suffering from venereal diseases. Musk melon should be taken for breakfast and also for dinner. The lunch should consist of cucumber, and bel-wood apple. The wood apple will take care of any costive tendency of musk melon. This diet may tend to weaken the patient but that should not be a matter of worry. After a fortnight of this diet, the patient can start on cereals, but only those which have been germinated, and then, they should form a part of the lunch: the breakfast and dinner should consist of fruits only. About 250 millilitres of cow's milk, boiled only once, can also be given at dinner time to the patient.

Initially the disease may seem intensifying when the patient starts on the diet mentioned above, but that need not cause any worry. Aggravation merely means that the system is trying to expel the poisons. Fasting can deal with the aggravation, if the patient can do it. Some of the energy of the body is utilised in digesting food and of the ingestion of food is stopped, that energy can be utilised to fight the disease by cleansing the blood. Enema must be taken regularly during the fasting period.

Mud bath is the other remedial procedure to deal with the sores and ulcers. Apply mud packs on the affected parts. Hip baths can also help speed up recoverey.

Nocturnal Emissions

Nocturnal emission or involuntary discharge of semen during sleep is one of the diseases which has given numerous quacks in cur country a golden opportunity to make money. A little excitement because of pornographic literature or seeing a hot motion picture may lead to night emission in a young man and if he is not properly educated about sex, he may be misguided into believing that it is a serious disorder. The belief is based on the traditional religious teaching in our country that semen is manufactured out of blood and that its loss is a disabling factor. Semen is, in fact, the fluid produced by the testicles and its emission during intercourse or in an involuntary discharge during sleep is not a serious disease as the quacks claim.

The person having such disorder should not get disheartened but take to clean, healthy living. Thoughts of sex should be avoided. They should not eat rich food in the mistaken belief that they must restore the energy lost through the loss of the seminal fluid. Rich food would merely give them a feeling of heaviness which will do no good. On the other hand, it is likely to disturb the digestive processes. The food should be simple and should consist of fruits, vegetables and a little of condiments. They should dine three hours before going to sleep.

Treatment

The person suffering from frequent night emissions must to get up early in the morning, go to the toilet, take a bath and go for a long walk. He should take a sunbath at about 7 a.m. His breakfast should consist of fruits and milk of cow, which should be boiled only once. His lunch should consist of chappaties made of wholemeal flour and boiled vegetables without any condiments except salt, turmeric and a little bit of cumminseed. A walk at about 5 p.m. and a bath later should be followed by an early dinner. He should go to bed at about 9 p.m. with a genital mud pack. This regimen is equally beneficial in hysteria, menstrual disorders or irregularities and frigidity in ladies.

Ejaculation (Premature)

Premature ejaculation is another disorder, which is also magnified by the quacks into something serious. It is only a malfunctioning due to psychological reasons. The male of the species is generally found to be sexually more aroused than the female who needs little time to get ready for intercourse. Too much of anticipation of the sex act, too much of excitement can lead to premature ejaculation giving a feeling of failure or lack of fulfilment which should follow the act of sexual intercourse. The only thing that can be recommended for this is to control one's feelings and not let the excitement get out of hand. A strengthening of the nervous system by following a regimen outlined under nocturnal emissions will also be highly beneficial.

Impotence

Inability to perform the sexual act is called impotance. It may be partial or complete, temporary or permanent.

The affiction is not very uncommon and can best be categorised into *organic* and *psychological*. Organic impotence may be caused by lesions of the external genitalia, e.g., a tight foreskin; disturbances of the endocrine glands such as diminished activity of the gonads, thyroid gland, or pituitary gland; diseases of the central nervous system such as locomotor ataxia (disordered movement of the limbs in walking); any severe disturbance of health as diabetes, addiction to alcohol, etc. Among the psychological factors which give rise to impotence are ignorance, fear, weak sexual desire, etc.

The only way to treat organic impotance is to deal with the disease which has caused it. If it is due to tightness of the foreskin, surgical help can be taken to free the glans penis or the folds of the prepuce. If alcoholism is the cause the patient must be advised to give it up and let nature clean his system of the alcoholic after-effects. In the case of glands being defective, they should be treated first.

In most of the cases the impotence is psychological. At the back of the mind of the person who complains of inability to perform the sexual act is a feeling of guilt which may have been engendered because of his having been addicted to masturbation in his adolescence or having fallen from his moral standards by indulging in incestuous or otherwise prohibited sexual relationships or some similar causes. It is the sense of guilt and shame which inhibits a person's performance with his wife. The feeling that he has over-indulged in sex may also cause this disorder. No physician has been able to define so far as to what is over-indulgence.

If hardly matters whether a person is guilty or not, but excess may lead to fatigue, both physical and nervous, and a temporary disinclination towards sex. That, of course, can be easily remedied, but the malady has to be tackled psychologically. The patient must understand that what he calls impotence may have suddenly arisen in his case. He should introspect and find the true reason. The moment he realises what has caused it, he is cured.

Treatment

The best treatment for impotence is a proper diet. Fruits, fresh seasonal vegetables—raw if possible, otherwise boiled—milk without boiling and germinated cereals should be the mainstay of the patient. Germinated grain is supposed to contain Vitamin E, the specific for impotence. The best germinated cereals are wheat, gram and the lentil *moong*. Soak them in water for 24 hours and then drain off the water but wrap the grains in a wet cloth. In another 24 hours the grain would germinate and ready to be eaten.

Start exercise; vigorous excercise. If you cannot run go for jogging but increase the distance of your jogging gradually.

Bask yourself in sun. Wear the minimum of clothing as you bath in sunlight. A wet pack on the spine can help ennervate the body by strengthening the nervous system. A bandage one-foot broad and two-foot long made of rough cloth—the best way would be a bedsheet folded into that shape—should be dipped in cold water and wrung. Spread that on a hard bed in such a manner that a part of the bandage overlaps the pillow. Lie naked on the bed so that the bandage remains in constant contact with your spinal column. Wrap yourself in a blanket. The coolness will percolate to your nervous system which is bunched around the spine and it will give you a feeling of peace and tranquillity. The cold bandage should be used for half an hour. Repeat it after lunch or during mid-day.

Consume water in adequate quantities: it will help expel all the morbid matter that has been poisoning your system.

The above-mentioned therapy is helpful in all sexual disorders, including night emissions.

Dysmenorrhoea

Dysmenorrhoea is such a complication which may vary from mere discomfort to an agonising colic, accompanied by prostration and vomiting. Sometimes painful menstruation as well as of stoppage of this function is caused by anaemia. Occasional pain, especially when it precedes the menstrual period, is due to irritation in ovary, and in this case it is generally accompanied by pain in the groin. For this type of pain, careful regulation of the bowels, regular exercise and the application of heat may prove to be highly beneficial.

Many women go through the agony of painful menstruation thinking this to be a normal condition. The maximum that they do is to take recourse to pain-killers.

The state of painful menstruation is an abnormal condition resulting from the wrong type of diet and an unnatural way of living. Too much of addiction to tea and pain killers to relieve the headache, addiction to refined and fried foods, lack of exercise—all these factors contribute to constipation in some cases of dysmenorrhoea. The chief cause of this malady is constipation and less than normal intake of water. Constipation is always at the root of pain. ful menstruation. The patient should give up refined foods, polished rice, sugar and potatoes. Food items like fruit and boiled vegetables, particularly greens with plenty of roughage, should be the mainstay of their diet. They will help relieve costiveness.

Amenorrhoea

This complication may surface due to anaemia, bad feeding, want of fresh air and all causes which depress the system, and cause loss of flesh, tend to cause diminution and finally stoppage of the menses. Diseases like malaria, aggravated dyspepsia, tuberculosis and sudden fright, great grief may also produce scanty menses or totally stop them. Excessive bleeding during menses may be due to a certain extent to the same general conditions which precipitate scanty discharge of blood. It is wellknown that the effect of sudden shock or deep grief on women has been observed to result in miscarriages and copious discharge of blood during the monthly periods. Besides that, the menstruation may start at an unscheduled time and may continue for longer periods than usual.

Treatment

In the breakfast the patient should have milk and fruit and her lunch and dinner should comprise of wholemeal bread, boiled vegetables with a lot of roughage and at least 2 to 3 litres of water in the day. Condiments and seasonings should be totally given up since they tend to produce acidity and increase costiveness.

The patient must start light exercise and go for walking regularly. It would be better if a hip bath is taken before one goes for a walk or takes exercise. The temperature of the water used for the hip bath must be 10° to 15° F. lower than the body temperature. Hip bath should be avoided during the menstrual flow, but might be taken if the pain is unbearable.

The exercises described below will help relieve all problems connected with menstruation, whether it is pain, their scantiness or profusion or even irregularity.

Exercises

Sit on the floor with your palms touching it and your legs extended outward. Try to raise your waist by putting all the pressure that you can exert on the heels of the feet. Repeat it at least ten times.

Lie on the floor with your arms parallel to your body. Lift one leg without lifting body: see that your trunk sticks to the floor. Then lift the other leg. Repeat ten times with each leg.

While lying on the floor, raise your body on your head and heels so that it is arched outwards. Resume the recumbent position and repeat this exercise ten times.

Put a pillow below your waist while lying on the floor. Fold your elbows so that your hands touch your chin. Raise your knees and extend your legs one by one. Repeat it ten times.

Avoid wearing high-heeled shoes and tight apparel.

The above mentioned regimen should be continued along with the diet suggested above till the patient is relieved of the symptoms which cause discomfort for her.

Leucorrhoea

Leucorrhoea is a symptom of many diseases peculiar to women. It consists of white watery discharge from the uterus. The discharge may be thick consisting mainly of pus, if the patient is suffering from a serious disorder of the genital organs, but in most cases it is catarrhal and chronic in nature. In mild cases, the discharge follows or precedes the menstrual flow but in more severe cases, it continues throughout the intervening period, Patients suffering from leucorrhoea look pale and unhealthy, get weary on the slightest exertion and a dull, gnawing pain is often experienced in the lower part of the back.

Cause of the disease, may be some infection, chronic inflammation of the womb following child-birth and gonorrhoea. The symptoms of leucorrhoea resemble those of nasal catarrh so much that it may be termed the catarrh of the womb. Both are marked by discharge of watery or thick humours and produce the typical symptoms of ill-health, like a pale face, loss of appetite, weakness and fatigue on the slightest exertion. Nature gives capacity to the diseased organ to expel the poisons from the system. That is why the naturopathic system has a similar remedy to deal with leucorrhoea.

The persons doing manual labour are least susceptible to colds and catarrh; similarly, women who do manual work do not easily fall victim to leucorrhoea. It is a problem of the indolent and ease-loving women who neither do any household work requiring the exercise of the body nor do any exercise.

Treatment

First of all, the patient must exercise her body by running, playing games like badmintion or tennis. The patients should reduce the cereals in their food and take to fruits and green vegetables diet as much as possible. Spices and condiments should be avoided as they tend to produce irritation in the membranes.

You will come across numerous eye catching advertisements of remedies about which tall claims are made. Such remedies may suppress the symptoms for some time but they cannot provide real or lasting relief. The only way is to lead a normal, natural life, in which the diet does not include refined, heavily spiced foods, Exercise of the body is essential.

The patient should take a bath, preferably in cold water, after she has taken exercise and then run her body dry with her palms. It will add a healthy glow to the skin.

The patient must avoid polished rice, and fish and meat as they tend to increase the mucus content of the humours of the body. Wholemeal flour and greens should form the major part of the diet. Vegetables, like carrots, tomatoes, onion, radishes, cucumber, spinach and other leafy edibles should be eaten raw. Milk and milk products should be avoided in the first two weeks of the treatment.

The patient should take a sun bath every day for fifteen to twenty minutes. During summer she may cover her head with a wet towel so that the heat does not harm her. She must sit in the sun till she start perspiring. Sipping warm water while sun bathing will help induce sweat. Bathe with cold water after sun bathing. In winter wash her hair with cold water and rub the rest of the body with a wet cloth dipped in cold water. Sun bathing should precede a meal by one hour or succeed it by two to three hours.

Cold compresses applied to the vagina can also help a lot. A cold compress may be worn like a sanitary towel for one hour or may be worn during sleep.

Menstruation (Delayed) and Anaemia

Anaemia can lead to delayed periods. Sometimes menstruation does not occur for many months at a stretch. One must take care of anaemia first. For that, raw vegetables, potatoes roasted in sand or over coals, cucumbers, tomatoes, carrots, leafy vegetables, spinach in uncooked form, oranges, pineapples, musk melons and mangoes should be mainstay. The patient should not take refined flour products, sugar and milled rice. Figs, dates, raisins and gur should be taken in place of sugar. Milk and milk products should be consumed as much as possible.

The patient should not overstram herself, mentally or physically.

Walking, exercise to improve the shape of the abdomen, sun bath in the morning and hot and cold hip baths can be of great help. Use tubs, one containing water at a temperature 8° to 10° degress higher than the body temperature and the other cold water. Alternate the tubs: five minutes in cold water and two minutes in the hot water tub. Repeat it four times and then take a cold bath.

Phosphaturia

The emission of phosphates with the urine is called phosphaturia. A whitish liquid precedes or follows the process of urination which is magnified by the quacks and the ignorant into a sexual disorder. The quacks make out that this is a vital fluid which is lost because of a sexual disorder or sexual weakness. It is nothing of the sort. Defective digestion can give rise to emission of phosphates, a vital group of minerals, along with the urine. If there are extraordinary emissions it is as best a deficiency disease and can be taken care of by toning up the digestive processes the naturopathic way. The regimen recommended for dyspepsia can deal effectively with this disorder.

Apprehension of Miscarriage

Pregnant lady feels any pain or there is slightest spotting (bleeding), She should take bedrest for three or four days. The foot of the bed should be kept raised a couple of inches for a few hours in the day when the patient is on bedrest. A wet pack should be placed on the pubes for an hour in the morning and evening both.

This therapy should be applied on the dates the pregnant woman would have had her monthly period. After the third month the apprehension of a miscarriage will recede.

Nausea among Pregnant Ladies

Constipation causes nausea among pregnant ladies. If they take care to see that constipation does not clog their intestines, they would not suffer from this complication.

Child-Birth in the Eighth Month

Natural salts, including calcium, are needed for the healthy growth of a child in the mother's womb. If the diet of pregnant lady lacks these salts, the foetus does not develop normally. The mother may suffer from atony or weakness of the muscles which support the uterus and may suffer a miscarriage and even if there is a normal birth, the child is most likely to be weak and sickly.

The pregnant lady should have leafy vegetables and milk in abundance. If an expectant mother takes a balanced diet and follows the principles of nature cure, she will bear healthy children.

Displacement of Uterus

In the womb uterus is slung in the pelvic cavity and has great freedom of movement upward, downwards, towards the right and to the left. Its natural position is for its long axis being directed upwards and forwards between the bladder and the rectum but the position at any time varies considerably according to the distension of the one or the other. Displacement of the uterus may occur because of many reasons and it is generally in inflammed condition due to displacement.

Downwards displacement of the uterus is known as prolapse and in this condition the uterus slips downwards in the space between the rectum and the bladder. Older women, generally face this condition, usually those who are becoming stout, have a considerable amount of the work to do and have in child-birth suffered laceration of the parts that should support the uterus.

Uterus distends during pregnancy when the foetus develops, its muscles getting distended along with the progress of the pregnancy. The muscles which support the uterus in its position must be strong to bear the load of the growing child. The stress on the muscles is very great during child-birth: they must have the capacity to support at least 15 pounds of weight. After delivery the uterus resumes its previous shape and the muscles resume their former size. In other words, the distension in the muscles is gone. If the tone of the muscles is missing, they cannot resume their original position.

Backache or headache, heaviness in the bowels and their costiveness are the symptoms which indicate displacement of the uterus. Some ligaments may become damaged and the mouth of the uterus may feel sore. The patient has the feeling that something is sticking to the uterus. Nerve centres are also badly affected due to the displacement of the uterus; the patient may be irritable and depressed. Sometimes there is fatigue and weariness which is felt all the time by the patient.

If the displacement causes too much discomfort the traditional physicians generally advise surgery. It consists of tying up the distended ligaments. Or a pessary might be fitted to keep the uterus in its right place. That is merely a palliative since the muscles which support the womb get some support, but they do not resume their former shape automatically. Surgical interference does not, of course, succeed and there may be many complications leading to constant pain and a feeling of unease which may persist all the time. Recovery after such an operation take quite some time. Unless the patient by lying in bed this complication may recur.

If the muscles in the body lose their tone or strength, their malfunctioning can result in such complications. Inactive muscles may also acquire a coat of fat and become unserviceable. Lack of proper exercise, acquisition of a coat of fat, deposition of morbid matter in the body and an inadequate diet lacking in essential vitamins and mineral substances can lead to atony of the muscles of a part of the body. A healthy female does not experience any difficulty in child-birth and there are no complications afterwards. Ante-natal care and proper diet can keep away the danger of displacement of the uterus.

Treatment

Naturopathy can efficiently deal with the displacement of the uterus. The more serious the displacement, the longer the period of recovery. If the patient is weak and old and her general health below average, it could take long to put her back in shape. Surgery may incapacitate the patient as a housewife for a period of a year or so, but naturopathy may take only a couple of months to give considerable relief to the patient.

Fasting is the first step in the treatment of such cases. Fasting should continue for at least three days. If a longer period of fasting is needed, it is better done under the supervision of a naturopath who would be able to take care of any emergencies that might arise due to this.

The next step is the improvement of the diet. It should include fruits, green vegetables and milk, milk products, refined food like sugar, and irritants like tea, coffee, sweetmeats and salt are not recommended.

For at least two weeks the patient should take bedrest, but must relax completely so that tension drains out of her body. She should lie on her back on the floor and take deep breaths. Then exhale slowly and try to relax her muscles.

Exercises

There are some exercises to tone up the muscles supporting the uterus. But before doing them, the patient should take a hip bath for fifteen to twenty minutes. The water level in the tub should be upto the navel. She should rub the parts, immersed in the water, with her hands vigorously. After coming out of the tub, she should rub the soaked parts with a rough towel and then start following exercises.

Lie on with face up on the floor and lift your legs alternately without bending your knees. After doing it for a few minutes, lift both the legs together. Then move the legs like pedalling a cycle.

Lift your waist as you lie with face up on the floor so that your body arches upwards, but your heels and the head should stay on the floor. Push out and push in your abdomen by deep breaths as you lie in that arched position. Repeat it for some minutes. Massage the abdomen first with the right hand, with circular motions upto the rib cage and then with the left hand.

Move your waist first towards the left and then the right as you lie in the position stated above. Your heels and your head should remain on the floor. Let your back touch the floor and then again arch your body upwards. Do this for ten to fifteen minutes to twenty minutes.

Lie on the floor with your face down. Keep your feet and the thighs on the floor, but raise your abdomen. Move it upward and downward for ten to fifteen minutes.

The patients will find it difficult to do these exercises in the beginning. Those with a protruding abdomen will find it more difficult. The purpose behind moving your abdomen up and down is to exercise the abdominal muscles and the thighs must not lose contact with the floor if those muscles are to be toned up.

Stand upright with your thighs touching each other and try to move your abdomen upwards by inhaling and contracting the muscles of the lower part of the abdomen. Loosen your muscles after each attempt.

In this exercise the patient should keep a hard pillow below her buttocks instead of under her head. Sleeping in this position, if that is possible, will help the uterus to return to its former position by the force of gravity. If you lie with your knees touching your breasts, that will also help the uterus to resume its previous position.

It would be much better if patient performs household chores in a sitting position. She should lie down after a meal with a pillow under her back.

If this regimen is followed for at least six months the patient will be highly benefited with it. One should not lose patience and always remember that the human body has wonderful resilience and atonic muscles can regain their strength with care, a proper diet and systematic exercises.

Constipation

This is a condition in which the bowels are expelled too seldom or incompletely. The patient may pass infrequent and hard, dry stools. The main symptom is the desire to void the stools but the inability to do so. It is an extremely irritating condition but easy to deal with if patient takes some precautions and go through systematic treatment.

This is a common problem and a large number of persons depend on laxatives to clear their bowels.

The persons who suffer from constipation do not understand the way the human body functions. It leads to many other symptoms like heaviness and headaches, lethargy, loss of appetite, insomnia and apathy. As a matter of fact, any disease is an indication of malfunctioning of the machine that is the human body.

If the body systems are unable to expel the waste matter that remains after the digestive organs have taken out the essential elements necessary for the sustenance of the human body, it leads to further putrification and gases harmful for their functions.

After the digestion process the food passes into the colon and that part of the body has a great capacity for absorption of liquids. If it loses its tone, that is if its muscles become weak or inactive, the stools have a tendency to adhere to it and continue to putrify leading to flatulence and other symptoms. Retention of stools could lead to poisoning of the whole system which leads to other serious complications.

When the laxative or purgative passes through the digestive tract, it produces new liquids which flush the colon and the stools adhering to it are voided in liquid form. But such substances are habit-forming and a chronic patient would gradually need more strong purgatives to clear bowels.

This is an unnatural and abnormal condition. Nature has endowed the intestines with the capacity to void the waste matter that remains after food has been digested. Hence, we must take the foods in their natural form. We pass the wheat through a sieve and polish the rice. We overboil the milk. Sugarcane juice is turned into sugar. We adulterate our foods with spices and condiments, which our body does not require.

Treatment

The patient should eat the wheat flour without passing it through a sieve; unmilled and unpolished rice is the best. Your food should contain two parts fruits and vegetables and one part cereals. Boil the milk only once, do not let it thicken by overboiling. That would give your food the roughage it needs and help the atonic muscles to void the waste matter.

If you are suffering from chronic constipation, eat more of tomatoes, carrots, spinach, cabbage and cucumber. The total intake of these should be a minimum of 250 grammes in the day. Eat them in the form of salad, season it with a pinch of salt and juice of a lemon in order to make it tasty.

You may eat three times in twenty-four hours, but if you are over forty, do not exceed two meals in the day. Do not take it literally: you can eat fruits in between the meals, but in reasonable quantities. It would be better if you would make fruits a part of your morning and evening meals. Talking of fruits, the best fruits are seasonal and those which are available to you within hours of having been plucked.

Constipation troubles some people, because their intake of water or liquids is too insufficient. The water intake should be three to four litres in summer and one to two litres in winter. A glass of water taken in the morning immediately after waking up can also be of great help.

The length of intestine is about 8.5 to 9 metres, it is in the form of one continuous tube suspended in loops in the abdominal cavity. At the lower end is large intestine through which your stools pass via the rectum. If the muscles of the large intestine lose their tone or strength, stools tend to adhere to its insides. Atony of the intestines can be cured by exercise. A walk in the morning or evening, jogging will also help a lot.

There is another way to void the stool is to cool intestine. Take a rough towel, fold it so that it can absorb water and place it on lower abdomen after immersing it in cold water. Let the coolness percolate to the abdomen for about fifteen minutes. A mud pack can also be used for this purpose. Take about one kilogramme of clay and knead it into a soft dough-like consistency and spread it evenly on your lower abdomen—from the navel to the pubes. Some people are known to have benefited more from a mud bath than from a cold towel. It should be done before you go for a walk. Cooling and then warming it through exercise helps the large intestine regain its tone in miraculous manner.

Initially you may not feel the urge to void your bowels. But do not wait for the urge. Visit the toilet at the time you usually do, even if the urge is not there. Remember that habit plays an important part. The best course would be to drink about half a litre of water and take a walk for ten to fifteen minutes before you visit the toilet immediately after dinner: it may surprise you to hear of intake of food followed by the effort to void your bowels, but remember that it takes fourteen to eighteen hours for the waste matter left after absorption of food into the system to leave the body. The churning of the stomach and the resultant activity of the intestines when you are ingesting food helps to give relief in constipation problem.

After forming the habit of visiting the toilet at an appointed hour in the morning and the evening, you will not have to spend more than four to five minutes there. In the beginning of the treatment suggested you may have spend a quarter of an hour in the toilet.

Patients facing problems like amnesia (loss of memory), constant insomnia, fatigue, incipient gout, asthma, indigestion, headache, lumbago and general weakness have found surease from these symptoms when they have regained the facility to void stools. A hip bath taken for five to ten minutes before they go for their constitutional in the morning or evening can help ameliorate their suffering caused by these complications.

Dysentery and Catarrh of the Intestines

Dysentery, results in inflammation and ulceration of the lower portion of the bowels. The chief symptom is colicky pain in the abdomen followed by diarrhoea, pain in the limbs and also fever. The stools contain mostly of mucus and blood. Bacillary dysentery has usually a sudden onset, whereas amoebic dysentery comes gradually leading to loss of weight and anaemia. In acute cases there may be perforation of the intestine and severe haemorrhage. Involvement of the liver generally results from chronic amoebic dysentery.

This complication called catarrh of intestines is a condition which worsens if not treated in the early stages. In a chronic state, it is generally less painful, though not less dangerous than most diseases. Whereas diseases like gout, asthma and eczema would cause pain in the chronic state, catarrh of the intestine is not marked by any pain or discomfort. Its chief indication is the passage of the mucus through the stools and a weakened condition of the patient. He would continue eating and drinking and unless he notices the mucus passing through the stools and takes some treatment, he loses weight, his aspect is wan and pallid and he feels lethargy.

The catarrh of intestines generally caused by chronic constipation. The large intestine, or the gut, through which waste matter is expelled from the body, has a spasm-like action which continues throughout the life. It takes the waste matter many hours to travel through the gut up to the rectum where it collects. A feeling of pressure is the signal from the brain to answer what is called the 'urge'. In a healthy body, the pressure is too strong to be withstood; if, however, it is ignored due to pressure of work, or other preoccupations the urge to void the stools becomes slack and the waste matter which should not stay in the gut for more than six to eight hours putrifies for 24 hours or even some days.

The function of intestine is to absorb the water content of the waste matter; if a malfunctioning of the gut leads to more than normal absorption, the stool becomes hard and dry. The gut absorbs the toxins along with the water from the waste matter which gives rise to morbid states. The hardness and a dry state of the stools leads to straining while evacuating them and nature compensates the friction which could harm the gut, by producing more mucus which is passed on with the stools. If this condition is not attended to in time, the inflammation may spread throughout the intestines. There may be perforation also which is a much more dangerous condition.

Treatment

The laxatives and purgatives taken to relieve the constipation merely aggravate the disease. Catarrh of the intestines takes many years to develop and its treatment in the natural way can take at least months: the patient should therefore, not lose patience. A start should be made with fasting. Only water, preferably lukewarm water, should, be taken. One should continue to fast as long as one is able to—four days to a week would suffice. Break the fast with clear soup of boiled vegetables without adding salt or any other seasoning. This should be continued for two-three days and then the patient should go to boiled vegetables, adding churned curd of cow's milk. The curd, churned and mixed with water, may consumed up to two litres in 24 hour.

To deal with the discharge of mucus with the stools warm water enema is recommended. Clay mixed with cold water may be plastered, over the lower abdomen up to half an hour. Mud pack can help deal with colic or dysentery.

A person suffering from catarrh of the intestines needs rest and fresh air. After he has gone through the regimen of a fast and then soup of boiled vegetables, he should preferably take vegetables, potatoes and plantains roasted over coals and curds. Cereals should be avoided as they tend to increase acidity. Salt should also be taken in small quantities and condiments, chillies and seasonings should be totally avoided. Fat, particularly oils, should be avoided. Butter can be taken in small quantities. Honey could be used for sweetening instead of sugar. The vegetables should be peeled off their outer covering before cooking. Fleaseed soaked in water may be taken twice in the day in the initial stages of the treatment.

In some chronic cases the curd treatment might be needed but complete rest is advised throughout the treatment. Light exercise, walking, might be advisable after some days of complete rest.

Catarrh of the intestines is an intractable disease and would need strong will power on the part of the patient to deal with. He must have faith and confidence that he would recover: not that without the faith and confidence his recovery would be hampered, it would only be slower. The greater the confidence and mental resilience of the patient will result in his quick recovery.

If someone drinks plenty of water, does exercises regularly and avoids heavily spiced, fried things, he is not likely to fall victim to the disease. The suppression of the urge to void bowels is the main culprit in many cases of catarrh of the intestines.

Indigestion or Dyspepsia

The basic digestive disorder is indigestion or dyspepsia which may give rise to more acute or serious diseases. The basic cause of indigestion, besides weak digestive powers, is over-eating or eating foods which must be avoided. Stools of such persons contain large amounts of undigested matter. They suffer from flatulence arising from putrifying matter in the stomach or the intestines. Belching may provide temporary relief, but there is generally a feeling of fullness amounting to heaviness, loss of appetite and general discomfort. Sometimes hyperacidity—presence of more acid in the stomach that is normal—may cause a burning sensation and even eructation (sudden escape of gas from the mouth or coming up of the undigested matter from the stomach). Overburdening of the stomach, the root cause of indigestion, must be avoided in such condition.

Treatment

The best remedy for dyspepsia is light food; it would be better if the patient takes to fasting for 24 hours and then takes to easily digestible, natural food. Fats and condiments must be avoided. Bland food, mostly vegetables cooked in water, juicy fruits and buttermilk (churned curd with water added) should be taken. Condiments and seasonings make food more palatable and there is the ever-present risk of over eating which is the root cause of dyspepsia. This is why bland food is recommended in this condition. Excess is bad and a person suffering from indigestion must eat less than he can digest. If he does so he can get rid of this problem.

If heat is applied through hot compresses or a hot water bottle to the abdomen for 15 to 20 minutes twice in the day, either on an empty stomach or two or three hours after meals, then it can activate digestive processes. The procedure could be alternated with cold compresses, applied for a minute or so in between hot compresses, could speed up recovery.

The above-mentioned procedure is merely a palliative. The patient can get permanent relief if he increases his body heat through vigorous exercise. Indigestion is the disease which troubles people leading sedentary lives, active and brisk people generally do not suffer from this complication. You may not be able to withstand the temptation of a second helping, but you can expend your energy through exercise which may be light in the beginning. Take a walk if you do not want to do vigorous exercise. Jog along if you can and walk on the dew covered grass will also be of great help.

Do not eat rice if you can, since rice is preferred with lentils which are not easy to digest. Eat rice with vegetables. Take fruits in-between the meals. Chew your food properly so that it mixes well with the saliva. Drink water in adequate quantity.

Use alcohol and tobacco in the minimum possible quantities, if you cannot give them up. If meat is taken it should be scraped down and should be free from fat.

Indigestion of a nervous origin which afflicts brain workers with sedentary habits can be treated on the lines indicated above. Such patients should, in addition to following the directions given above, consciously avoid thinking about their condition and should try to remain happy. A change of scene and climate is also recommended.

Worms

Our intestines are sometimes infested by parasites which trouble us greatly. The most common parasites in India are: tapeworm, hookworm, roundworm and the threadworm. They exist in the intestines because they find a congenial climate for their growth which again is the result of wrong type of feeding which most people indulge in. Patients suffering from these worms generally acquire a voracious appetite, but in spite of massive quantities of food they take, they do not gain weight. Sometimes they are pale and sickly and, therefore, gloomy. Infants and young children are likely to be irritated all the time and are prone to throw tantrums at the slightest chance.

The threadworm is the least harmful and most common parasite. When they are expelled from the anus, they tend to create uncontrollable itch and the patient is forced to scratch his anus. They are small, thread-like creatures which can be noticed in the stools of children. The hookworm and the tapeworm resemble earthworms: they are less common in our country than threadworms.

The root causes of this problem are bad habits like eating food without washing hands, putting the finger first in the nostril then in the mouth, eating contaminated food, scratching the anus and then eating food without thoroughly washing the hands, using underwear worn by a person suffering from threadworms, constipation, and mucus in there stools, which invite the parasites to infest the intestines.

Treatment

There are many drugs to kill the parasites; they may give temporary relief, but that is more likely to harm the digestive processes and create other complications. Nature care, on the other hand, aims at strengthening the intestines so that they can purge themselves of the parasites. The stools of a child suspected to be suffering from threadworms could be examined visually: in some cases they would be found sticking to the anus of the child.

Start treatment of theadworm infested patient with cleanliness. A child suffering from it should be administered a warm water enema to which juice of half a fresh lime should be added. It should be followed by administration of about 50 to 100 millilitres of coconut oil with the help of a syringe through the anus. The child should be asked to strain himself at the time of visiting the toilet.

It would be much better if the treatment is started with fasting: if the young patient or his mother cavils at it, he should be administered fruit juice or clear vegetable soup mixed with water. Lukewarm enema must be given during the treatment both in the morning and evening. Enema would help expel mucus and threadworms from the intestines. Bed clothes of the patient must be aired in the sun every day and he should be kept in an airy room.

In case if the child is walking he should be encouraged to fast for two days followed by a diet of fruits and boiled vegetables for five to six days. Raw vegetables like carrot, cucumber and onions can be given in addition to tomatoes. Milk and cereals should be totally avoided. Potatoes roasted over the coals and raisins soaked in water could also be given. After that the patient could be allowed porridge or gruel. When he has started taking cereals, milk should not be given to him, but do not give him lentils.

Mud pack and cold compresses applied from the navel to the pubes can also help in the initial stages of the treatment. Juice of garlic could also be taken recourse to since it kills the parasites without causing any harm to the patient.

The same regimen could help in dealing with diseases like hepatitis, enlargement of the spleen, low fever, prolapsus of the rectum, goitre, mumps, swollen eyes in children and discharge of pus from the ear.

Ulcers and Hyperacidity

Hyperacidity: If the hydrochloric acid present in the stomach increases in quantity, the condition is known as hyperacidity. It is this condition which gives rise to gastritis (inflammation of the mucous membrane of the stomach) and ulcers—gastric, peptic and duodenal. Almost all these diseases present some difficulty in diagnosis because of confused symptoms, unless there is a bleeding ulcer. Generally the symptoms of dyspepsia appear in above mentioned complications.

Ulcers: The main cause of ulcers is dietetic indiscretion, like ingestion of heavy meals, addiction to alcohol and smoking. Food poisoning, infections like influenza, septicaemia and toxins like uramia and gout are the other causes of gastritis and ulcers. The mucous membrane of the stomach gets congested and too much of acid gives rise to wounds or ulcers. The size of the ulcer is from ¼ to 1 inch in diameter, and it is either round or of an oval form. It tends to penetrate through the abdomen.

The indications of ulceration in the stomach are dizziness, nausea, eructation and loss of appetite. Acidity goes on increasing leading to a burning sensation or even pain in the stomach which is relieved after ingestion of food. As the disease progresses there is distension of the stomach due to excessive flatulence, mental tension, insomnia,bad temper and gradual weakening of the body. Constipation also appears and sometimes the traces of blood can be noticed in stools of the patient.

Serious problems like haemorrhage, perforation and obstruction of the pylorus (the orifice through which food passes from the stomach to the intestine) also arise. Unless it is detected in time massive bleeding may lead to death. Traditional medicine has recourse to blood transfusions in an emergency but there is nothing else it can do in such a condition.

Besides dietetic indiscretions, habits of thought also play a vital role in cases of ulcers. Those given to excessive anger, tension, jealousy, worry and hurrying are more exposed to the malady.

Allopaths also recommend bland food free from acidity and condiments for ulcer patients, but they generally overlook the psychological aspects of the disease. They advise the ulcer patients alkaline diets or drugs containing alkali, but that is not anything more than a palliative.

Treatment

The patients having ulcer should avoid spices and seasoned or fried foods. Nothing that is likely to augment the acidity of the stomach should be consumed. Alcohol is, forbidden in ulcers. Cream, butter, milk, fruits and boiled vegetables are the best diet for an ulcer patient. The fruits recommended are mangoes, musk melon, banana and dates. This regimen would progressively reduce the acidity in the stomach of the patient.

In chronic cases the patient should take only milk and fruits. Milk should be taken in moderate quantities—say about 250 to 300 millilitres—every hour. Leafy vegetables should be avoided in the beginning. The various types of gourds should be boiled without their rind because the rind is likely to create friction in the stomach. Flea-seed husk—10 to 15 grammes—should be taken with water or milk after every meal.

The ulcer patient must drink one to one and a half litres of water during the day. He must bathe in cold water twice daily. Hip bath for ten to fifteen minutes and clay plastered over the lower abdomen for half an hour in the day can help the ulcers to heal. The hip bath or the mud pack should be taken on an empty stomach and should be followed by a walk. In case of constipation, daily enema should be taken.

Regular massage and deep breathing exercises also help. The patient must also try to get rid of his worries and stay cheerful. It has to be remembered that hyperacidity does not come up suddenly: It is a gradual development and its cure is also a gradual process. If the patient does not lose patience and continues the regimen suggested, he can get rid of his problem.

Dilation or Distention

This is associated with hyperacidity it is another disease of the stomach: distension or dilation. It can occur without giving rise to any symptoms. If food is retained for a long time in the stomach, it gives rise to fermentation. The condition is both painful and irritating. It also take its toll on the health of the patient.

In this condition also, the only hope is the naturopathic way of controlling your diet. The regimen suggested for ulcers and hyperacidity can help in this complication.

Flatulence

In some cases excessive wind is formed in the stomach. There is a rumbling sound issuing from the insides a couple of hours after meals. The sound is so loud that even other people can notice it.

This rumbling sound after ingestion of food indicates a state of putrifaction in the stomach and the intestines. It indicates over-eating and bad digestion. People who gulp down their food generally suffer from this malady. One must chew the food properly. If one eats sweet, sour and refined foods one is merely inviting trouble. One should take natural foods: breakfast on fruits and boiled vegetables in lunch.

Have a cup of hot water half an hour before meals. Exercising abdomen muscles and walking can help in ameliorating the state.

Enlarged Liver

This is a common problem among children at the age of nine or ten months and they start getting weaker and weaker. Though they are breast-fed at this stage, then why they suffer from this complication? The reason is that the mothers of such infants subsist on cereals, ghee and sugar alone. They should take more milk, vegetables and fruits to be ables to produce healthy milk for their baby.

Diabetes

Diabetes, is a disorder of assimilation. When the pancreases become inactive or atrophied and cease to produce insulin, the body is unable to convert the sugar into energy for the muscles. Its chief symptoms are weakness and loss of weight, great thirst and increase in the amount of urine passed. There is sometimes voracious appetite but the patient gradually becomes more and more emaciated. Owing to poor vitality of the tissues, various skin eruptions like boils and carbuncles appear. There may be itching in the groins and eczema. A serious complication could be gangrene of the skin of the feet, beginning with the toes. A curious phenomenon is that the younger the patient, the more rapid is the course of the complication.

Allopaths administer insulin to dissolve the sugar in the blood and forbidding starchy and sugary foods to the patients. Modern science has not been able to pinpoint the real cause of the disease: what is available is only generalisations such as, fat persons are more susceptible to the disease, it attacks males more than females, or that it is hereditary, etc.

Treatment

In this condition also the Nature Cure recommends a diet and no drugs. The main purpose is to help the body to assimilate the sugar into the system and that can be achieved by a special diet. Some experts commend about one kilogramme of curd made from cow's milk and various types of gourds without salt. The greener the vegetable, the most beneficial it would be. Sour fruits like oranges, pineapple, tomato, rose apple (*jamun*), could also be taken with advantage. The patient can also take one or two chappaties made of flour which has not been passed through sieve. The person suffering from diabetes must go for long walks (preferably eight kilometres) daily. Remember that the disease strikes generally those who lead a sedantry life, and fond of rich food.

Sugar, sugar preparations and cereals should not be taken for some time. The other method of treating the disease is by fasting for a couple of days and then eating sour fruit only for a week during which green vegetables may also be alternated with the fruits. Curd made from cow's milk must form an inevitable part of every meal. If the curd is not available, about 50 grammes of germinated gram, may be taken with every meal. After about a fortnight of this regimen, the patient can take bread made of whole flour. During the period of fasting, lukewarm enema should be taken daily.

The patient must do physical exercise as that helps to utilise the blood sugar. Walking, preferably jogging, is the best exercise for them. Hip bath is extremely beneficial in the case of diabetes, particularly for patients suffering from constipation. For a leathery skin most diabetics develop, the best exercise is vigorous rubbing of the skin with a rough towel for fifteen minutes before a bath with cold water.

Most of the physicians while recommending a sugar-free diet to the diabetic, prescribe a high protein diet like fish, eggs, meat and lentils leading to an imbalance in his food. Advising patients to take saccharine instead of sugar, the allopaths expose them to the danger of slow poisoning. The harmful effects of saccharine have come into notice by recent researches.

The patient must also try to remain happy and keep his poise.

Hernia

Protrusion of any organ, or part of an organ, into or through the wall of the cavity which contains it is called hernia. The most common form of hernia is the hernia of bowel, popularly known as rupture.

This complication may be caused due to a defect or injury of the abdominal wall or increase of pressure within the cavity. It may be caused by sudden exertion as during the lifting of a weight, but generally it develops gradually. Pain may be experienced while coughing or straining at stool, but really acute pain is suffered when a hernia becomes strangulated as the result of stoppage of its circulation by the pressure of the opening through which it protrudes. It may become inflamed, turn acutely painful and may even produce peritonitis—inflammation of the membrane lining the abdominal cavity—and finally prove fatal. Stoppage of the bowels, onset of acute pain and vomiting are the ominous symptoms which indicate strangulated hernia.

More males than females suffer from iguinal hernia—where the iguinal canal, through which the testicles descend, gets blocked—and more women from femoral hernia because of the shape and inclination of their pelvic bones.

Treatment

The allopaths prefer surgery to cure a hernia. The covering through which the hernia protrudes is stitched after the hernia has been pushed back to its proper place. But experience has shown many fatalities a couple of weeks after the surgeon has done his best. And then, surgery does not succeed. The offending hernia appears again and again in spite of surgical aid.

The truss—a pad of lint or folded handkerchief kept in position by a spica bandage—is a mere palliative and never a cure. The best treatment according to naturopathy is exercise. The torn muscles, the site of the hernia could be helped regain their tone and strength by application of the cold compresses or application of bandages covered with soft clay. Compresses should be continued for half an hour at a time and should be applied twice or thrice in a day. Diet plays an important part in dealing with a hernia as it does in other diseases. The patient should take light, bland food, comprising boiled vegetables and fruits in order to reduce the pressure on the intestine. Too much of weight of waste matter would merely burden in increasing the danger of worsening the problem.

The wearing of a truss can help during the treatment of the hernia. It comprises a pad which fits over the opening a spring to run round the pelvis and a strap to pass between the legs and prevent the truss from sliding upwards. Special trusses can be made by firms manufacturing medical and surgical supplies according to the needs of individual patients. The patient must find the truss which suits his hernia. It should be worn constantly so that the hernia does not recur. The regimen suggested should be followed strictly get cured.

Exercises for Hernia Patient

(1) Lie straight (face up) and fold your knees to touch your abdomen. Then straighten them slowly without lowering them on the bed.

(2) Hold the bed with your hands and raise your legs and try to touch your head with your feet.

(3) Raise your feet perpendicularly and then twist your legs, first to the right and then to the left. Turn more towards the direction opposite to the site of the hernia.

(4) Lie on a hard bed and make somebody hold your feet firmly or bind them with a strap passed round the end of the bed. Put your hands on your waist and raise your head about six inches. Turn left and then right and resume your previous position.

(5) Lie in the position as above and put your arms behind your neck. Then try to raise with your feet in the previous position. But do not overstrain yourself.

Prolapsus of Rectum

Prolapsus of the rectum is common among children. Generally, people do not pay sufficient attention to children's health. Dried stool due to constipation force a child to strain too much and the rectum is displaced from its natural position. Such children must be asked to visit the toilet at fixed timings in the morning and evening and should be made to take water in adequate quantities. The diet of the children should be such that they should not face constipation problem.

A clay pack applied to the rectum for half an hour thrice or four times daily can deal with the prolapsus of the affected part.

Milk for Atony of Intestines

There are people with weak intestines and they suffer from fevers which continue for long periods. Doctors who examine them tell that they might even get TB of the intestines. One loses weight and have night emissions too due to this complication.

One should start a milk diet to strengthen the intestines; that will deal with night emissions and also add to the body weight. Live on orange juice for three days taken in quantities of 200 to 250 millilitres taken three to four times in the day. A daily enema is essential. On the fourth day take to cow's milk. The first day's diet should be 250 millilitres of milk taken at one hourly intervals. Reduce the interval to 50 minutes the next day and then to 45 minutes till on the sixth day the interval should be only 30 minutes. Continue the milk (250 millilitres at 30-minute intervals) for one to one and a half month. The drinking of milk can continue from six in the morning to six o'clock in the evening. The total quantity will be about six litres, but that will not be much and cannot harm the digestion. The best way is to take the milk without boiling; during summer it can be stored in refrigerator.

If somebody suffers from constipation from a milk diet, he should not be afraid; an enema will take care of it. If it leads to diarrhoea, discontinue it for some days and take churned curds instead. The curds should not be stale and the cream which will appear on it when churned should be separated. Stop separating the cream after six or seven days.

If one gets bored of taking nothing but milk, he can suck a lime. In a diet of churned curds, drink some orange juice after each feed.

Have a sun bath for 15 minutes in the morning and a bath with water at body temperature at about ten in the morning. During the course of the milk diet, take rest at short intervals.

After following regimen about one and a half month gradually reduce the quantity of milk, by taking it only up to 1 p.m. and then switching on to fruits in the evening with half a litre of milk. On the third day when one has stopped taking milk in the later part of the day, he may start a diet of boiled vegetables and bread in the evening. He may take water when he feels like.

After completion of the treatment, one can take to normal exercise in the morning and evening with usual diet.

Piles

This complication is a varicose and often inflamed condition of the veins about the lower end of the bowel. Haemorrhoids are either external, internal or mixed. In external piles there is not much bleeding but a lot of pain, whereas the internal piles consist in discharge of several ounces of dark, thick blood.

This is not a disease in the strictest sense of the term but a symptom. It is caused primarily by constipation. The pressure applied in voiding a constipated bowel tends to distend the veins and the external piles may be swollen causing pain making it difficult for the patient to sit. The piles get enlarged and red and give off a thin, blood-stained discharge.

Most of the allopaths recommend surgery than drugs in the case of intractable piles, but even removal of the offending part does not give relief since the disease is likely to recur. Piles is one disease about which a lot of fuss is made: you would come across a lot of nostrums and indigenous drugs to get rid of this problem.

Treatment

Treat first of all the basic cause and that is constipation. The use of violent and irritating purgatives should be avoided and care must be taken to secure soft motions. The nature cure way is to regulate the diet. The diet of a person suffering from piles should be a little different from the one recommended for dealing with constipation. Some haemorrhoid patients become allergic to some foods even if they tend to relieve constipation. The best diet of secure a soft stool, the instrument of relieving constipated bowels, will comprise wheat porridge, whole meal (wheat flour without being passed through a sieve), green vegetables, particularly spinach, gourds of the various varieties, cabbage, radish, fruits like ripe banana, papaya, musk melon, apple, pear and milk. Lentils and *daals* should be avoided since they tend to cause constipation. Dry fruits like figs, raisins, coconuts are also recommended. The best regimen for the piles patient could be to breakfast on papaya, or musk melon and milk. For lunch he should have porridge and leafy vegetables and his dinner should consist of: (a) some vegetables and raisins, (b) vegetables, figs and currants in addition to some bread, or (c) coconut and fruits or cooked vegetables in medium quantities. Dry fruits like currants, raisin and figs could be taken up to 200 grams at one time, but the best way is to soak them in about 400 millilitres of water and take them along with the water. Flesh of fresh coconut could be taken up to 125 grams and dry coconut up to 75 grams at a time.

The above-mentioned regimen will give relief in most of the cases, but in chronic or intractable cases where the patient passes dry, hard stool aggravating his condition flea seed (Isbagol) is recommended. Flea seed or its husk should be taken in small quantities of five to ten grams. The best way is to soak it in water, 20 times its volume for 24 hours and take it before every meal. The quantity should be reduced when the condition gets better.

The people suffering from piles are generally drink less water than demand of their bodies. They must drink 2 to 3 litres of water in a day.

The clay therapy can also benefit the patient. Take 1 to 1½ kilograms of dry clay and knead it into soft doughlike consistency. Spread it like plaster from the naval to the pubes; a ball of clay should be kept on the rectum for half an hour. The mud treatment should best be taken one and a half to two hours before breakfast and repeated before dinner. After the mud is removed, a brisk walk for three to four kilometres will be highly beneficial.

If above regimen does not work, then the patient should take resort to fasting. Fasting should last from three to seven days, during which nothing but water should be taken. It would be difficult to do it in the beginning and the patient should try it for three days in the first instance. Lukewarm water enema must be taken in the morning or evening during fasting. And a fasting patient should return to normal diet only gradually, starting with vegetable or fruit juices, going on to porridge and milk and then to normal food.

Fever

Most of the physicians blame germs as the causative factor in fevers and its practitioners talk of incubation periods, viruses and other organism. The main factor, however, is the predisposition of the body towards diseases, whether it is fever or pain. If that were not so, all persons exposed to an infection should get infected.

According to nature cure fever develops in a body only when the system is in a condition of internal uncleanliness. Fever is a direct manifestation of an acute disease but at the same time it represents the effort of the body to expel the poisons which have accumulated in it. If the fever is allowed to run its course in a natural manner, the sufferer would be in better health than before after the body has thrown off the affliction. Body systems themselves are capable of cleaning the body.

Physicians cure the fever with drugs but it succeed only in suppressing it. There may be a seeming cure after the administration of drugs and the temperature may go down but in umpteen cases maladies more serious than fever result because the drugs suppress the ejection of the poisons which nature tried to by means of a rise in the temperature of the body. Most of the chronic diseases can be traced to the suppression of acute disorders by the use of medicines.

The fever is a natural crisis and it must be helped to run its normal course; any interference, such as administration of drugs, is only likely to retain the poisons which caused the crisis. The first thing that should be done to help the body to carry out the spring-cleaning is to make the sufferer fast. The system of a person suffering from fever does not need any food because all his energies are directed towards ejecting the poisons accumulated in the body. If the body has to divert a part of those energies towards the digestion of food which in most cases is forced on the patient because the well wishers think that his strength is to be maintained, the only result is that the course of nature is obstructed creating complications. One must not forget that anorexia—loss of appetite—accompanying most fevers is a signal from nature that patient should not be given anything to eat. Allopaths adopt the procedure in the matter of typhoid fever but fail to understand that it is the only method to take care of all kinds of fevers.

Treatment

The storage poisons in the body, which results in fever, can be dealt with by making the patient fast. Only water and orange juice in limited quantities should be given to him. The patient must avoid food for a week. Only when the temperature has dropped to 98° F and the tongue of the patient is a healthy pink only then he should have his normal diet.

During the fasting period the patient should be given a warm water enema daily; it should be discontinued after he has started having his normal diet.

To reduce temperature of the body cold packs are safe and best: they may be applied to the whole of the body in the case of high temperatures like those of malaria and typhoid, and to the throat in the case of diphtheria, to the chest in pneumonia.

Take a large piece of linen material or a sheet dip it in water, wrung it and wrap twice round the body (in the case of high temperature) and cover patient with a blanket. The pack on the throat should be covered with a piece of flannel. Cold or tepid sponging of the body is also recommended and if the patient can stand it he may be given a cold shower. The packs may be removed after temperature has come down to 100° F but the body should be thoroughly sponged. Mud-packs and hip baths are also beneficial.

When the temperature has gone down and the tongue of the patient is no longer furred, he should be put on an exclusive fruit diet for some days. The first two days only juice of fruits should be given and then the whole fruits: oranges, grapes and other juicy fruits are the best. On the third day a limited quantity of unboiled fresh milk can be added to the diet of the patient. After he has been on a diet of fruit juices and milk for three to four days, he should be advised to start taking boiled vegetables and unleavened bread made of whole meal. If fruits are not available during the period of convalescence, vegetable juices may be given. Non-vegetarian soup should be avoided by the patient.

There are other diseases of which a fever is a cardinal symptom. Any special precautions to be taken in the case of the various maladies are discussed under the appropriate headings. Even though the fevers dealt with here are of the more serious variety and all the categories have not been discussed the regimen indicated would help in other fevers also.

No matter whatever the disease is, if there is fever, it should be treated first, because if it is properly handled, the poisons which gave rise to that disease will be expelled through the fever. After the fever has gone down the virulence of the disease of which it was a symptom will be reduced considerably; it is just possible that the disease may vanish with the fever.

Influenza

This is an acute disease similar to all other fevers. Its cardinal symptoms are: high temperature, aches over the whole of the body, stiffness of the limbs and a sore throat.

Though the fever in influenza is not very high it rarely going above 103° F, but its seriousness consists in its aftermath when serious complications in the form of infection of the lungs or the respiratory tract occurs. If broncho-pneumonia develops after or during the last stage of influenza the poison may spread to the heart and cause cyanosis which may result in death.

Though experts blame a virus or an epidemic for influenza, the real cause of its development is the toxic and run down condition of the body. It originates through a lowering of the vitality of the individual. It is interesting to note that most influenza epidemics have started and do start during or just after winter. Sometimes, it strikes people at the junction of the seasons. Like all other diseases it is a natural attempt of the body to clean itself. If any complications arise in a case of influenza it is because of the wrong type of medicine which aims at suppressing the disorder. If it is treated like an ordinary fever, there is no danger of any kind.

Treatment

Influenza should also be treated like all other fevers with a minor difference, viz, fasting should be undertaken for five to seven days depending upon the elevation of temperature of the body. After the fast, the patient should be kept on an all-fruit diet for a couple of days. Milk and fruits may be allowed thereafter followed by boiled vegetables.

Malaria

This is common in tropical and sub-tropical regions, particularly, places which are moist and dirty. The causative parasite enters the blood stream through the bite of a mosquito of a particular variety. Most of the physicians use quinine and its derivatives for treating malaria.

Initially, the patient has vague pains all over the body, headache and a slight rise of temperature. The onset of fever is preceded by a feeling of chilliness in the hottest of weather and no amount of blankets or quilts gives any relief from the chill. With the rise of temperature, the hot stage begins when the fever may reach 106° F or even more. After several hours of high temperature, the sweating begins and the fever comes down leaving the patient extremely weak and emaciated. The fever may come again the next day, two days later or even after three days.

Treatment

The most popular remedy for malaria, as has been mentioned above, is quinine, but a large number of cases develop complications like loss of hearing, anorexia and a feeling of unease. In some cases the parasite may not be found in the blood and may lodge itself in the spleen or the liver making the case more complicated.

Malaria should be dealt in with the same manner as all other acute fevers. If the temperature goes beyond 105° F the body of the patient should be wrapped in a sheet dipped in a iced water to bring down the fever. The moment the temperature comes down to 102° F the iced water routine should be discontinued.

Milk should never be given to the patient. Loss of appetite is a natural concomitant of malaria, it's nature way of warning the system not to take anything. Water should be given freely and in extreme cases of weakness. fruit juice—preferably that of orange—may be given in moderate quantities.

If temperature during intermittent malaria comes down, it should not be taken as an indication of complete recovery of the patient. He should continue to fast till the danger of reappearance of the fever is past. If after the temperature has gone down, there is a feeling of chill, the patient should be given a hot hip bath. Alternatively, he should be advised to take hot water bottles to deal with the chill.

Measles

This is a contagious disease of children—it rarely strikes adults, but if it does, it leaves them prostrated for quite some time—more common in warm than in cold weather. It begins with a slight feverishness, cold in the head, running of the eyes, and dry cough. On the fourth day from the onset of the malady, a rash appears on the body. It is noticed first on the face and the neck. After five days of rash when the fever continues to haunt the patient. it starts peeling off. The patient feels drowsy and confused and is very touchy. Diarrhoea sometimes appears but, generally, nine days after the onset of the disease, the patient gets well, the temperature goes down to normal and the appearance of the body resumes its original condition.

Treatment

In this complication medicine should be administered after the appearance of rash. In naturopathic treatment fasting is recommended, the child may be given only orange juice and water to drink and no milk at all. Measles weakens the eye tissues and the child should be kept in an airy, semi-darkened room so that sunlight does not harm the eyes. When the fever is down and the temperature comes back to normal, the child should be kept on an all fruit diet for at least three days. Only when he has thrown off the effects of the malady and his tongue is clear, he may have normal diet.

Chicken-Pox

This is usually an infantile disorder: it rarely attacks adults, but when it does, it leaves the patient prostrated for quite some time. There is fever and a skin eruption in the form of vesicles which look like blisters. They dry slowly and scabs are formed. The vesicles appear in crops; as one batch dries up, another appears as opposed to small-pox where the vesicles develop simultaneously over the entire body.

Treatment

Fasting is the first step in the treatment of chicken-pox. Only fresh orange juice and water should be allowed to the patient with an enema morning and evening till the temperature comes down to normal, the scabs over the vesicles fall and the tongue reattains its healthy hue. The eyes of the patient should be protected from strong light as it is likely to harm the tissues. If there is cough present along with the fever in the earlier stages of the disease, cold packs to the chest should be applied to relieve the condition. The patient should never scratch the vesicles.

Small-Pox

This is an acute infectious disease which has taken a huge toll of human lives in the past. It is only recently that it has been wiped out. The orthodox treatment for small-pox is mainly preventive. Inoculating everybody has had the effect of pushing the dreaded scourge into the limbo of history. But cases are extant when the disease has been caught by persons inoculated. Sometimes inoculation has had deleterious effect on the health of the person.

This disease launches sudden attack without any premonitory symptoms. The temperature suddenly shooting upto 104° F or more with shivering; the pulse is rapid, extreme thirst, pain in the back of the neck, intense headache and vomiting. There is an eruption, more serious than that of scarlet fever, all over the body. The vesicles resemble blisters which harden and later on fill with pus. They dry up, the scabs fall off but they leave ugly scars on the body. In severe cases the eruption appears also in the eyes, making a person totally blind.

Treatment

There are two sides to the treatment of this dreaded disease: preventive and curative. Prevention consists in keeping the environment clean and a clean, healthy living according to the principles of naturopathy. If fever of small-pox strikes, the treatment is the same as in other fevers. The best way to deal with the eruptions on the body is to keep them clean; the patient should be prevented from scratching himself as he has the temptation to do because of itch which comes on during the period when the scabs are falling. Scratching will only delay the recovery and the pitting on the skin may be more pronounced. A little olive oil should be heated and applied with a swab over the scabs. That will not only alleviate the itch, but would also help the scabs to fall soon.

The patient suffering from small-pox should be given a cold sponge twice or three times a day. Alternatively, the parts of his body on which there are no vesicles, should be wiped with a piece of cotton-wool dipped in cold water.

Typhoid Fever

This is a condition in which there is an insidious fever, a typical course of temperature, marked abdominal symptoms consisting of ulceration of the bowels, an eruption on the skin, an uncertain duration and a liability to frequent relapses.

The initial attack of the fever is milder than most fevers. The patient may go about his work for a week or so till the progress of the disease confines him to bed. The most marked early symptoms are lassitude, headache, a general discomfort, insomnia and feverishness, particularly at night. In some cases there may be nose-bleed in the early stages. The fever rises in the evening and has a tendency to fall in the morning: the temperature of typhoid is typical. Each succeeding day the highest and the lowest point tends to increase till the disease has run its course. Skin eruptions tend to appear in the second week and if care is not taken inflammation of the bones and ulceration of the bowels may occur. Exhaustion leads to prostration. Ulceration of the bowels may lead to haemorrhage and if an ulcer is perforated, peritonitis may set in with fatal results. Sometimes inflammation of the lungs or the pleura leading to pleurisy—may result and the patient, even though free from fever may be confined to bed for months.

This complication invades only that body in which there is accumulation of toxic waste and other putrifying materials in the intestines. If a system is healthy and free from toxicity there is no likelihood of typhoid developing, even if the person is exposed to the severest form of infection.

Treatment

The physician has a tendency to wait for a complete diagnosis before proper medication and by that time the disease has taken hold. The best way is the way of nature cure where a fever—no matter what its name and variety—is treated by same methods.

The sufferer must take to fasting till the temperature goes down to normal. During this period only water and orange juice in medium quantities should be given to him. After the fever is gone and the tongue has regained its healthy pink colour, an all-fruit diet should be given followed by boiled vegetable and un-refined foods like unpolished rice and wholemeal bread.

Rheumatic Fever

Rheumatic fever means rheumatism accompanied by rise in temperature and pain in the joints. It is a serious disorder of childhood which has a tendency to involve the heart. Modern medicine believes it to be the result of what is known as streptococcal infection and is treated with massive doses of penicillin. Infection of the tonsils caused by the organism sometimes precedes the onset of rheumatic fever. Lack of a particular hormone leads to disturbance of the tissues. But what modern medicine fails to explain is how the lack of that hormone takes place.

Its initial symptoms are chilliness or rigors, followed by feverishness and a feeling of stiffness or pain in one or more joints, generally those of the larger size, such as the knee, ankle, wrist or the shoulder. The temperature goes up to 103° F, the pulse is rapid, the tongue is coated and there is loss of appetite and constipation. The attack may pass off in a few days, but it returns with increased vigour and if it becomes chronic, the inflammation of the membrane, the outer covering or the muscle of the heart, may develop leading to serious consequences. Sometimes, the temperature rises beyond 106° F endangering the life of the sufferer.

This fever is usually confined to children and adolescents; among adults it usually assumes a chronic form. If a child complains of pain in his joints, it should not be ignored because more often than not, the pain is an indication of rheumatic fever.

The root cause of this disease is over-eating of acid forming foods; the daily ingestion of meat and demineralised starchs, refined sugar, fats and other unnatural edibles flood the human system with impurities which cause the rheumatic fever.

Treatment

The treatment is the same as in other fevers, namely, fasting and keeping the patient on orange juice and water with a daily enema. In addition, cold packs should be applied to the swollen and aching joints. Whole body packs may also be applied if the fever rises beyond 106° F as it is likely to.

Scarlet Fever

This fever is characterised by high temperature of the body, a sore throat, and a diffused red rash all over the skin of the body. Modern medicine believes the fever is caused by an infection to which children are particularly susceptible. The onset of the fever is sudden, the temperature rising to 104° F in a few hours with the skin eruptions beginning to appear within 24 hours. It takes about a week to subside. A serious complication that may arise is the inflammation of the kidneys particularly during the period when the patient is convalescing. The fever may return and the kidneys may refuse to function resulting in stoppage of urine and consequent uraemia.

Scarlet fever is a volcanic form of spring cleaning that nature undertakes in certain cases. As in other diseases, the predisposition caused by bad eating habit is the real culprit.

Treatment

Its treatment is same as indicated in other fevers. When the rash of scarlet fever starts peeling—and the process is likely to continue three weeks after the temperature goes down to normal—epsom salts bath, twice or thrice in a week will ensure quick recovery.

In case epsom salt is unavailable, common salt can be used in its place. A kilogramme of common salt should be put in a tubful of water the temperature of which should be 102° to 104° F. The patient should be made to lie in it for half an hour. He should be given a glass of cold water to drink before he gets into the bath and a cold towel should be used to wrap his head. Such a bath is also useful in cases of rheumatism when there is no fever.

Pneumonia

Pneumonia is the inflammation of the substance of the lungs which manifests itself in many forms. The attack usually commences with shivering (in young children, convulsions), followed by pain in the chest and sometimes vomiting. The temperature rises suddenly to 104° F and the pulse is extremely rapid. The breathing is shallow and laboured. There is a dry, hacking cough. If there is expectoration of phlegm, it is rusty. The fever is usually between 103° F and 105° F for about a week when it may fall suddenly. There is profuse sweating at the time and the pain may abate as the disease intensifies.

Children are more often than not its victims even though the disease may strike any person of any age. Pneumonia is sometimes a complication resulting from a inappropriate treatment of influenza.

Treatment

This complication among children is often the result of suppressive medical treatment of other diseases of a less serious nature. Its treatment according to naturopathic principles follows the same lines as for other fevers. The child suffering from pneumonia should be fasted for several days—during that period only water and fruit juice in medium quantities should be given. No milk should be given. Packs to the chest will help relieve the condition. A daily warm water enema should be given. It may have to be repeated 3 to 4 times during the day according to the need.

Meningitis

This is a term applied to inflammation of the membranes of the brain or the spinal cord. It generally strikes children, though adults may also fall victim to it.

Initially the patient becomes listless and fatigued, suffers from headache after exertion and irritability. After that comes vomiting and an obstinate constipation. In some cases the first symptoms are convulsions. Headache is extremely severe and there is great intolerance to light. Then there is the rigidity of the neck and of the lower limbs. The temperature rarely goes beyong 103° but the pulse does not rise proportionately. It does, however, exhibit some-irregularity. The second stage of the malady is a state of depression, which is sometimes taken to be a sign of improvement. But, in fact, it is a condition of apathy or partial stupor. Vomiting and fever are less severe and the former, sometimes vanishes totally. The third and the final stage is that of paralysis in which fever returns. The pupils are dilated and there may be complete loss of sight and even hearing. During a fit or seizure when the body is convulsed the death takes patient in its grip.

Treatment

It should be treated in the same manner as all other fevers are treated but it is better to leave the patient in the case of a competent naturopath. Fasting, wet packs and warm water enemas will all have to be given according to the condition of the patient. An all-fruit diet is recommended when the fever goes down and normal feeding should not be started before the sufferer has completely recovered from the malady.

Diphtheria

The initial attack of diphtheria is mild, with a low fever and soreness of the throat. A membrane appears on one of the tonsils and continues to grow. It is surrounded by a zone of inflammation. The glands of the neck are usually enlarged. The child is extremely weak and if the poison of the diseases reaches the heart there is little hope for the patient. The malady is ascribed to some germs and the doctors talk of incubation periods, all children do not get it even if they come in contact with infection. Proneness to the disease is the major causative factor. Wrong feeding, unhygienic living and continued constipation are the real culprits. Modern medicine has developed a serum or anti-toxin to prevent diphtheria but cases are on record where the administration of the serum has led to many serious side-effects. The serum sometimes suppresses the helpful bacteria and the toxins and impurities which the system was trying to expel.

Treatment

Fasting is the first step in the treatment of diphtheria. No milk should be given to the patient. Warm water enema must be given twice daily. The child must lie on one side and not on his back so that he does not swallow the secretions from the infected tonsils. Absorbant cotton balls may be placed in the mouth to absorb the secretions. Cold packs should be applied to the throat at two-hourly intervals and if the fever goes high a cold pack must be applied on the whole body.

In this complication after several hours of a high temperature, the sweating begins and the fever comes down leaving the patient extremely weak and emaciated. The fever may come again, the next day, two days later or even after three days.

Whooping Cough

A whooping cough patient should give up all foods which produce phlegm like ghee, sweets, milk, rice, refined flour products, lentils and sugar. His diet should consist of oranges, musk melon, tomatoes and raspberry. Vegetables like spinach, cabbage, gourds, should be taken in a boiled form without addition of any condiments. Wholemeal bread and roasted potatoes could also be given. The patient should be advised to fast for a couple of days with the onset of the symptoms of whooping cough. The fasting period should be followed by a week of living on oranges only. See to it that the child does not develop costiveness.

Discharge of Phlegm

This complication troubles those who consume refined flour, milled rice lentils and milk. Vegetables and fruit can reduce the amount of phlegm produced in the body. If the food is not properly digested or assimilated by the body, phlegm is abnormally high. Exercise and increasing of the vegetable contents of the food would deal with this condition.

Drinking of warm water about a litre with a tablespoonful of salt mixed in it can give quick results. Drink it after you have gone to the toilet and then vomit it out. Most of the phlegm would be expelled.

Common Cold

It can be called coryza or catarrh of the nose, a common cold is a very irritating condition. It may be caused by a variety of factors, the most common being a sudden chilling because of a change of temperature, coming out of a warm bed into a blast of cold breeze or walking from an air-cooled room into a blazing sun. These are only predisposing factors, the real culprit being a virus, which incidentally has not yet been separated or counteracted. Traditional remedies fail to cure the cold. But in the case of weak constitutions a cold may lead to more serious diseases like laryngitis, bronchitis, pneumonia, tonsillitis and tuberculosis. What is worse, a catarrh of the respiratory organs may degenerate into a catarrh of the alimentary system.

A cold is an extremely irritating one is not sick enough to get into bed, yet not well enough to lead a normal life. A running nose, feverishness, heaviness of the head, pains and aches in the body, loss of appetite and of smell are the main features of a cold which makes life miserable of the sufferer.

Treatment

Cold is also the result of inappropriate diet. It is nature's way of expelling poisonous humours from the body. The malady must be attacked at its source and that is the putrifying matter in the intestines. The patient must fast till the cold is gone. It will not last more than two days and take a warm water enema followed by a cup of warm water after every two hours. If he is unable to take the enema, then he must try the following method.

Take half a kilogramme of spinach, 250 grammes of turnips (along with their leaves), 250 grammes of tomatoes, 75 grammes of coriander leaves and 25 grammes of ginger. Cut them into small pieces and boil them in about one litre of water. If some of these vegetables are not available, radishes or other greens may be used. Cover the lid of the vessel with a flat dish full of water so that the water does not evaporate and there is sufficient left. When the vegetables are done, strain them through muslin or other fine cloth. Add a little salt, the juice of a lime and roasted and ground cuminseed and take it in tumblerfuls after every two to three hours. This will clear the bowels and also open the pores by inducing perspiration.

Sometimes a cold becomes chronic. Such patients should also follow the regimen suggested above. It will clear their bowels. They should also do some exercise so that their pores open. Those who are too weak should soak their feet in warm water for fifteen to twenty minutes before going to bed at night. The patient must wear a blanket while he is doing it; it will help open his pores and stop nose running.

Sore Throat

This is usually the result of a chill. Milk and milk products are harmful in such a condition. The patient should have a glass of lukewarm water with a spoonful of honey in the morning and before sleep at night. Apply a cold compress to the throat and cover the compress with a woollen colth. For a week he should take bread, fruits and vegetables only.

Asthma

This is a disorder of the respiratory system characterised by severe paroxysms of difficult breathing. The onset of an attack is sudden, though the patient starts feeling uneasy, drowsy and irritable a little before the difficulty of breathing starts. Respiration becomes difficult and the breath comes with a wheezing and sometimes whistling sound. The general belief is that asthma is a chronic disease and that once gotten continues to dog its victim till the day he dies. Allopaths say that it is due to allergy in most cases and that when the causes are removed, the patient will be relieved of this malady.

Naturopaths say that asthma is caused by excess of phlegm and the inability of the body to expel it. If the patient gives up food which tend to increase the phlegm, e.g. rice, flour passed through a sieve, sugar lentils, milk and curds, he can find relief. He should be put on foods which discourage phlegm, such as green vegetables, fruits, and the like. That would tend to reduce the amount of phlegm present in the body and the disease will leave him. Unfortunately, under the false impression that asthma being a weakening disease, the patients are fed on high protein diets like eggs, meat, fish, milk and milk products and fats and that worsen their condition.

Treatment

A patient suffering from asthma must select foods which help contain the amount of phlegm in the body. For breakfast he should take foods like orange, tomato, papaya, guava, mango and rose apple and vegetables, like carrots. His dinner and lunch should consist of boiled vegetables. His bath is recommended in the morning and evening to perk up his digestive powers. Taking a walk is also recommended, if he is unable to do jogging.

During its severe attacks, asthma tends to destroy the appetite of the patient. He should not be forced to eat. He should keep fasting till the attack is over. The only thing he should take is a cup of warm water every two hours. An enema taken at that time would be doubly beneficial. If this regimen is followed, the attack will not last for more than 36 hours and the chances of a recurrence would be remote.

The patient should take to regular fasting once a week and take an enema the morning after the fast to clear his bowels. If he is unable to fast regularly, he must not hesitate to stop eating the moment the attack comes. A fortnight after the treatment has been started the patient can take cow's unboiled milk or curd with a breakfast of fruits.

The asthma patient should be extremely careful in his eating habits. He must never overeat. The amount of food taken at one time should be so measured that he must feel extremely hungry at the time of the next meal. A salt-free diet would be extremely beneficial for him.

At the time of asthmatic attack, soaking of the feet in warm water can relieve the agony to a great extent. A chest pack can also help, even though on application it may seem to aggravate the attack. The pack applied in the afternoon and immediately before, sleep would do wonders. The main aim of treatment of asthma should be to augment the vital force of the body with the help of proper diet and natural living in which clean water and sunlight play a vital role.

The above-mentioned regimen is helpful in the treatment of tonsillitis also.

Bronchitis

The inflammation of the tubes that lead from the throat to the lungs is called bronchitis. The inflammation tends to impede the process of breathing because phlegm tends to stick to its insides. The treatment outlined in the section on asthma should help in bronchitis too, but the following procedures are being repeated here once again with slight changes.

Treatment

The patient must take to fasting as long as the acute symptoms last. He should only take water and orange juice. An all fruit diet should be taken when the fever attendant upon bronchitis has gone down and the breathing is easier. A hot epsom salt bath every night or alternative nights will be beneficial during the acute stage of the disease. A wet pack should be applied to the upper part of the chest every day. Towels dipped in hot water and wrung out applied to the chest are also helpful. The phlegm sticking to the insides of the bronchial tubes will be dislodged and the sufferer will feel an immediate relief in breathing. After the hot compresses, a cold compress should be applied to achieve the desired result.

After recovery the sufferer should start normal diet because if that is not done, the disease is likely to recur and it may become chronic. Breathing exercise, a friction sponge (rubbing the body with a hand-towel dipped in water and wrung out) should be taken regularly. Hot epsom salt baths should be taken twice or thrice in a week.

Tuberculosis

This is one of the most dreaded diseases which has troubled mankind for centuries and is caused by the organism *mycobacterium tuberculosis*. It may affect any part of the body, but the most important form is the TB of the lungs. The severity of the disease depends on the organ involved. If it affects the membrane of the brain, it causes what is known as meningitis. Its manifestations are inflammation of the bones and the swelling of the joints. If it attacks the glands of the body it is called scorfula. Bones, the intestines and the genito-urinary tracts are also the sites of this killer disease resulting in death in many cases.

In initial stages there is cough of an irritating nature, particularly in the morning. The first major sign is the spitting of blood. There is loss of appetite, colour and strength followed by emaciation and loss of weight. A very important sign is a regular rise in temperature, either in the forenoon, or more often in the early afternoon, with a fall below normal in the early morning. The digestion processes are thrown out of gear—diarrhoea or constipation can also be noticed. There may also be pain in the chest indicating the involvement of the pleura. The second stage begins when ragged cavities are formed in the lungs; X-ray examination shows effusion and the symptoms described above become more acute. In the terminal stage, the lung shows signs of shrinking and sometimes, it falls in. If the throat becomes involved, the voice is husky, the diarrhoea becomes more troublesome and there may even be haemorrhages. Emaciation is now extreme, the temperature swings from one extreme to another and there is copious sweating. Death comes due to excessive loss of blood or sudden lowering of temperature and the inability of the lungs to suck air efficiently.

As per naturopathy, the main causative factor in TB. is the devitalisation of the system because of wrong feeding and a lowering of the vital force. Mineral starvation of the tissues of the body as a whole is the real culprit. Colds, catarrh and malaria, if suppressed, may also make way for tuberculosis.

Treatment

Treatment for this fatal disease is to have the patient stay in clean, healthy surroundings where there is plenty of fresh air and sunlight. The germs that cause TB die quickly if they are exposed to direct sunlight than if they are boiled. It is a disease of filth and poverty and proper steps should be taken to keep the environment clean. Once it strikes a person he should be first treated for fever as indicated in the section on fevers. Cold packs to the chest and throat should be applied twice to thrice daily till the temperature comes down to normal. Spitting of blood should not frighten the patient since that is the way of nature to get rid of the poisons accumulated in the body. No so-called nourishing food as meat broth or milk should be given so long as the temperature of the body remains above normal. Only orange juice and water is to be given and a warm water enema to get rid of the poisons in the intestinal tract. Fresh fruit diet should be started when the temperature has become normal and milk after 3 to 5 days and should be continued for some weeks. The intake of milk may be increased gradually. TB is generally associated with depletion of natural calcium in the body and milk is the best source of that calcium. But milk must be taken unboiled and fresh.

A sponge bath is also recommended in the morning and breathing exercises should be started. A hot epsom salt bath is also recommended. The diet—after the fever has subsided—should consist of vegetables, milk, fruits, wholemeal bread, butter, eggs, cheese and nuts. These foods are the richest in organic calcium and would aid recovery. All devitalised foods like refined wheat flour, sugar, tinned and preserved foods should be given up.

Tonsillitis

Tonsils are two almond shaped glands situated at either side of the narrow passage where the mouth joins the throat. They have the structure of lymphatic glands and consist of an elevation of the mucous membrane of the mouth presenting twelve to fifteen openings. Even though at one time it was believed that they did not play any vital role and could be excised when infected, but researhes established their importance as a guard against infection. The children whose tonsils had been removed were more susceptible to infections than others. The tonsils act as a fishing net, trapping most of the infections and localising them.

The attack of tonsillitis is sudden, with pain in swallowing and sensation of chilliness and fever. The swelling is caused by harmful bacteria and poisonous substances which enter through the food. One or both tonsils become enlarged and are covered with a varying amount of whitish or grey material, which is a purulent discharge from the tonsils themselves. Sometimes the pain travels to the ear. The tongue, particularly the posterior part, is covered with a thick fur, and the breath has an unpleasant odour. The temperature of the patient sometimes rises to 104° or 105° F.

Tonsillitis is generally preceded by coryza. Wheat bread, rice and potatoes generally tend to aggravate the predisposition towards the disease, but the main cause is the bodily poisons. Cold, dyspepsia, loss of sleep and constipation are some of the predisposing conditions of this malady.

The causes of this complication are many, like overeating, consumption of whitened foods like refined sugar, addiction to fried delicacies, condiments, conventionally cooked vegetables, tea and coffee are only some of them. Predominance of these substances increases acidity and alkalinity is diminished. Refined bread may give the calories, but it lacks in essential vitamins and minerals which are extremely essential.

Most of the people prefer foods which produce constipation and that is the root of most of the bodily disorders which afflict them, the reason being that the poisonous matter is not expelled from the body, as it should be. They do not breathe deeply and do not let the lungs do their proper work, nor do they take fresh air which inhibits the pores in the skin from exuding poisonous humours through sweat.

Treatment

A patient generally loses his appetite: it is nature's way of safeguarding the health, or at any rate, from letting it deteriorate further. The best way to deal with the disease is to stop taking solids: the patient should only take juice of oranges, lime and honey, and of course, water. An enema should be taken daily so that all waste matter is expelled from the systems.

Secondly, patient should avoid foods which produce or increase acidity. A bath in lukewarm water, better still having cold and hot baths alternatively helps. Saline gargles or gargles with lukewarm water mixed with a few drops of fresh lime juice can also help. Chest and throat packs should also be resorted to. Massaging the neck and the backbone can help reduce the severity of the attack.

Cold and hot baths taken alternately and rubbing of the skin vigorously with a damp cloth can help the skin too to eject the poisonous humours. Rub the skin till it glows: that will enervate the skin and increase its capacity to resist disease.

After few days when the acute attack has subsided, the patient should be kept on fruits alone. When his condition improves he could be permitted to take salads and boiled vegetables. Tea and coffee, sugar and refined flour products should be prohibited. Deep breathing and exercise could increase the oxygenation of the blood and the patient would recover quickly.

Body Itch

This is a skin disease caused by impure blood. The best way to purify the blood is to ensure that you void your stools and pass urine in adequate quantities and also perspire so that poisonous humours are expelled from the body. Take an enema daily to clear your bowels, take as much water as you can and spend some time in covering your body with a cold bandage. What you should do is this: spread four blankets on a hard bed or on the floor. Take a cotton bed sheet, dip it in cold water and wring it lightly. Spread the wet sheet over the blankets. Take off your clothes and lie down on the sheet, covering your body with it. Wrap the blankets over you one by one. Within half an hour to one hour you will perspire profusely. Drink some hot water before you wrap yourself in the wet sheet and the process of perspiration will be hastened. After an hour take a cold bath. Take this treatment thrice in a week. On alternate days, rub your skin with your palms after wetting them with cold water. The pores will open and expel harmful humours.

A salt-free diet is recommended in itch, the patient can start having salt after he is cured. He should have tomatoes and green gram for lunch and bread and green vegetables for dinner. In case green gram is not available, eat germinated gram.

Light paste of coconut oil and lime juice can be applied on itching skin. That will destroy the germs that cause the itch. Itch is contagious, hence, keep away from other people.

Eczema

Eczema is one of the most common diseases of skin, it consists of an inflammation of the skin of a catarrhal character. It is attended with papules, vesicles or pustules, attended with more or less discharge, and with itching and other symptoms of irritation. It is, in fact, a symptom denoting the reaction of the skin to various forms of irritation. It is generally found in persons of morbid constitution where the excretions of the bowels or kidneys are not up to the mark.

This complication when in its acute form, shows itself by redness and swelling of the skin, the formation of minute vesicles and severe heat and irritation. If the vesicles rupture, a raw, moist surface is formed, from which a colourless discharge oozes, which forms skin crusts when it accumulates. Such attacks may occur as a result of digestive derangements, or in persons of rheumatic or gouty tendency and they tend to appear at certain seasons, such as spring time.

The eczema may be dry, weeping or rubrum where it affects only the leg. Administration of drugs has only a palliative or temporary effect. Homeopaths believe that the suppression of eczema may produce symptoms of more serious diseases since, according to them, it is the result of psoric poisons. The real cause is the failure of the human system to excrete the poisons from the various orifices of the body. Waste matter is excreted from the rectum, through the stools, from the bladder through the urine, from the breath through the lungs and from the pores of the skin. The pores are an important outlet from which poisonous humours are discharged through sweat. The condition of the skin is a very good pointer to the state of the health. Sometimes the pores of the skin are over-worked since the person does not expel the waste matter properly from the other orifices. That is why the perspiration of some persons is rancid: it may even smell of urine in few cases.

Treatment

If the systems which expel the waste matter from the body perform efficiently, if the bowels are clean, water is taken in sufficient quantities, the urine is clear, the lungs are able to breathe clean, fresh air, the skin will remain healthy. If the pores of the skin are not given the chance to perform their given functions properly, the sweat is full of morbid humours which give rise to the various skin diseases, like eczema, acne, boils, and other eruptions and itch.Trying to cure an eczema by skin applications is not justified. In such condition the relief is temporary. If the exudation is suppressed, it may be a prelude to some other more serious complications.

The first step to treat eczema is to cleanse the blood and the body. The sufferer should get as much of fresh air as possible. The people who live of narrow airless streets in a city slum should migrate to the open areas of the villages and let fresh air cleanse their system. Tight clothing should be avoided if one is suffering from eczema.

The patient must drink two to three litres of water daily and must bathe twice to thrice in the day. The skin should be vigorously rubbed with the palms of the hands before taking a bath. All the parts of the body should be thoroughly wetted and rubbed to such an extent that the towel is not needed to dry the skin. The site of the eczema should, of course, be spared the rubbing.

Bathing in a lake or a river, is also beneficial, but do not dry yourself with a towel. Lie on the sand or take a walk so that the water dries in the sun. Take another bath; alternate your bath with the sunbath. If this is done at least twice in a week, it will help a lot. The area affected by eczema should be covered with coconut oil. It will help the skin to stay soft.

The patient must take an enema if a diet of fruit and fresh vegetables does not help relieve his constipation. Walking or jogging should be resorted to in order to activate the bowels. He must walk at the rate of six kilometres per hour for at least two hours daily.

Our blood is alkaline and so are fruits and green vegetables. They are most suitable for us and should be consumed in adequate quantities. Cereals, sugar, salt, fats and boiled milk add to acidity and should be avoided if possible. Onions, garlic, radish should not be consumed.

The treatment should start with one week of fruits and vegetables. Salt-free boiled vegetables with whole meal flour is recommended after one week's fruit fast. Coconut oil may be used instead of ghee. After some time curd and milk could be consumed.

Musk melon and carrot are particularly beneficial in cases of eczema. They should be taken three to four times daily reducing the intake later on and adding milk and curds. Musk melon should be washed down with cow's milk. The combination of musk melon and milk is not harmful as it is believed.

Besides that, the sunlight is also a nature's scavanger: it kills all the harmful bacteria. Sunbathing should be done early in the morning, in the first light of dawn. Stand or sit in the sun till you perspire: if it is too hot, cover your head with a wet towel. After you have perspired, take a cold bath.

A light mud pack applied over the site of the eczema is also helpful in dealing with it. The pack should be allowed to remain for one hour at a time; it could be repeated twice or their in the day. A mud pack over the whole body dried in the sun and later washed with cold water could be highly beneficial.

In chronic and more difficult cases of eczema the patient should be advised to fast at least one day in the week till he is cured. One week's fasting could cut down the recovery time considerably. Prolonged fasting must, however, be undertaken under the guidance and supervision of an efficient naturopath since it may raise certain problems for a layman.

This complication as a by-product of dyspepsia, gout or diabetes could be cured only after those diseases have been successfully treated. Children suffering from eczema as a result of insanitary bottle feeds can get relief if kept on fruit juices or water with a teaspoon of honey mixed in it.

Acne

This is a skin disease affecting the sebaceous gland (glands which produce an oily secretion). These glands are especially large upon the nose where their openings form pits that are clearly visible. There appears to be an individual predisposition to the disease and is dependent on the development of the sebaceous glands which takes place at puberty. It occurs in both sexes particularly between the ages of fourteen and twenty. The condition is often associated with dyspepsia, and lack of fresh air and exercise. In women it tends to become worse during their menstruation period.

The eruption itself consists of little black spots which indicate the mouth of small sebaceous ducts chocked with dust or dirt, from which a long, wormy-looking fatty mass can be squeezed; hard pimples generally showing one of these blackheads on the top; little pustules surrounded by a slight degree of inflammation, which gradually grow, burst and then heal; and hard lumps, sometimes half an inch in diameter which last for weeks or months, slowly suppurate and leave a permanent scar on the skin.

Acne is the sorrow of the beauty-conscious female and a medium of providing bread and butter to the drug manufacturers. There are numerous lotions, creams and drugs claiming to cure acne. Such remedies cannot cure acne, of course, but are bought at great expense. The only thing that they do is to suppress the action of the sebaceous glands temporarily. Blemishes left by the removal of black heads can only be hidden under a coat of make-up, which tends to worsen the condition of the skin by clogging the pores.

Treatment

Acne are the result of dyspepsia and constipation which must be treated before there can be any hope of dealing with acne. The surest cure is to improve the diet which must not contain any sugar or fat as it tends to increase acidity and hence dyspepsia and constipation. Hygiene of the whole body must be looked after properly and a lot of fresh air and exercise taken to reactivate the pores to expel the poisons from the body through profuse perspiration.

You must include fruits and vegetables in your diet. Take plenty of exercise and lots of water so that your bladder ejects the morbid matter through its activity. Seasonal fruits and raw vegetables like tomatoes, carrot. cucumber, spinach and cabbage should be your mainstay. If this dietary regimen is continued for some months. acne would disappear.

Steaming face can also be of great help. Take boiling water in a basin and hold your face over it so that the steam opens the pores. After about 15 minutes of this treatment, wipe the face and wash it in cold water. Dip a swab of cotton in fresh juice of lime and rub it on your face gently. Let the juice dry on the face and then wash it after some time. It will not only remove the dirt that might have gone into your pores but would also give it a glow of freshness to the skin.

Leathery Skin

In some cases the skin turns leathery during winter and develops a blackish crust; the onset of summer automatically brings improvement. The reason is that the perspiration during winters is much less as compared to the summers, which means that the pores exude much less morbid humours than they do in summers. Do vigorous exercises to produce sweating. Also see that a major part of your diet consists of fruits and vegetables.

Crow's Feet and Loosening of Face Skin

In some cases the skin of face hangs in folds and there are crow's feet under the eyes.

First of all, the person facing such problem must improve his health by following the principles outlined in this book. Secondly, he must have an optimistic outlook on life. He should drink at least one to two litres of water daily.

The sufferer must wash the face and neck with warm water and then give it a cold douche. He should not wipe the skin with a towel but massage it with the palms. The palms must move upward from the neck. He should sesame or coconut oil over the face and neck before going to sleep: pat the face lightly after application of oil for three to four minutes. Wipe the oil with a soft cloth and then with a wet towel. The anger and irritation add to the lines of age on the face, so one should avoid them. A smile, better still, a hearty laugh exercises the muscles of the face better than anything and that can take care of the loose skin better than any other remedy.

Kibes

Some persons suffer from kibes during winter. The hard crust on the heels cracks and starts bleeding. It is not only painful but incapacitating condition for them. But in summer the kibes heal on their own.

This complication is caused by lack of alkalinity in the

blood and also unclean feet. Take more vegetables and fruits to make up the deficiency of alkaline matter in the blood and wash your feet scrubbing the heels thoroughly. Wash the feet with hot water and apply coconut oil on the kibes.

The sufferer should wear shoes; walking barefoot will not only make the feet dirty but the dirt will get into the cracks of the heels because of the kibes and create further problems.

Boils of Face (After Shave)

In some cases boils appear on face after shaving. When they burst the pus spreads and so do the boils. They also cause irritation.

A close shave sometimes produces small boils on the face. One must make it sure that the razor is clean. A cold compress on the face while going to sleep can help. Foment the face with a hot compress two or three times in a day, but wash your face with cold water after a hot compress. They will activate the circulation of blood. Also take a sun bath for a quarter of an hour in the morning. An exclusive diet of fruit for three to four days, with a daily enema, will speed up the recovery.

White Spots on Nails

White spots on the nails indicate calcium deficiency. Take leafy vegetables and milk in adequate quantities; the white spots will be replaced by a healthy glow on the nails.

Some particular serious diseases are associated with partial loss of hair as one of their symptoms. They are: acute fevers, myxoedema (degenerative conditions of the subcutaneous and connective tissues due to a defect in the thyroid gland), syphilis, influenza, anaemia and great anxiety or severe shock. Gradual premature baldness is generally hereditary. Sometimes it is preceded by dandruff which, in its turn, is caused by decomposition of the natural oil in the hair. Each day in the process of combing, a certain number of hair which have reached the end of their existence, fall out and are replaced. But, if the change is too rapid, baldness is inevitable.

Falling of Hair

If the hair fall out as a result of any particular disease, they are likely to be replaced when the patient gets rid of the disease. The hair may, in that sense, be called a barometer of disease. The moment the falling of the hair is noticed, one should take to vigorous massage of the scalp, because, if the hair fall and a fine down appears on the scalp, it means that total baldness is unavoidable.

The hair band or the cap should never be tight because it is likely to interfere with circulation of the blood in the scalp.

Massage the scalp thoroughly and vigorously, rinse the hair with cold water and then comb your hair. A cold douche of the hair is always helpful if done regularly. The best way to do it is to immerse your head in a flat-bottomed vessel for a minute. The hair should be combed with the fingers and dried through massaging.

Water is not harmful for the hair as is commonly supposed. The best way to take care of your hair is to wet them thoroughly with water and then to vigorously rub the scalp.

The emergence of dandruff is a morbid condition of scalp, which is caused by the excessive secretion of the sebaceous glands. The secretion mixed with dirt forms scales or a distinct encrustation. It can interfere with the nutriment reaching the hair and also to baldness. Dandruff is infectious and personal articles like comb, towel, etc. of the patient should not be used by others. The hair of the patient should be cut short and the scalp kept clean. The hair should be washed with whey, gram flour and myrobalan soaked in water.

Some people think that it is caused by the disturbance of the sympathetic nervous system. The real cause, however, is the disturbance caused in the veins carrying blood to the skin. That is why the affected skin turns pale and rough. The only remedy is a vigorous massage of the affected part. No applications of any oils or creams have had any marked effect once the disease launches its attack.

Lice-Infested Hair

Lice-infested hair due to the insanitary condition of the hair. The hair may be cleaned, but what of the lack of sanitation in the body? Women should take to a diet of fruits and vegetables for some weeks. They should also wash the hair with a decoction of myrobalan, whey or juice of lemon mixed in lukewarm water.

Grey Hair

Hair turn grey with age but sudden shock may also produce the effect. The colour of the hair should not concern one of their health. Darkening agents should be avoided as they contain substances harmful for the skin. In cases of premature greying, open air exercise, massage of the scalp, dietary regimen, particularly ingestion of raw vegetables, is beneficial.

Eye Care

The health and the beauty of the eyes depend on cleanliness of the body. Constipation, for example, makes the eyes dirty. The white of the eyes no longer remains white; inadequate intake of water may give them a yellow tinge. Insufficient perspiration gives rise to accumulation of poisonous humours in the body and dark circles appear around the eyes. Smoking also gives yellowish colour to eyes.

The inner cleanliness is the key to the beauty of the eyes. Improve your diet, enjoy sun-shine and fresh air. Spend at least 15 to 20 minutes in the sun with the minimum of clothing so that fresh air can get into your pores and the heat of the sun can induce perspiration.

The food must have all the necessary vitamins. Vitamin A is to be found in abundant quantities in carrots, leaves of turnip, sweet potatoes, milk, butter, cabbage, tomatoes, peas, gourds and spinach.

Vitamin B can be found in the husk of the soyabeans, wheat, milk, peas, unpolished rice, toasted rice, raisin, cucumber, oranges, spinach, carrot, cabbage and pineapple.

Vitamin C can be found in green chillies, juice of lime, orange, leaves and stalk of the mustard plant, spinach, leaves of turnip, papaya, leaves of beetroot plant, tomato, cabbage, mangoes and myrobalan.

The most economical sources of natural Vitamin D are: milk, butter and sunlight.

Exercises

Fold your arms with your hands under the armpits and stand in a relaxed manner. Take your shoulders back in a circular motion and resume the previous position.

Touch the underside of the neck with your chin and then move your head as far back as you can. Move your head in a circular motion so that it touches first the right and then the left shoulder. Then move in the reverse direction touching first the left and then the right shoulder.

Move your head from side to side without moving your body. Keep your head stationary and then move your eyes upward and then downwards. Move your eyes left and right. Repeat this process at least six times.

Fix your gaze on your index finger extended outward and try to view a distant object across it just as you are taking aim. Repeat it twenty times.

Stand with your feet one foot from other. Close your eyes and move your body from right to left. This should be done facing the early morning sun. Sprinkle cold water over your eyes and then dry them with a soft cloth.

Put your palms on your eyes. Sit with your elbows on your knees and palms on your closed eyes. Do it softly so that no pressure is exercised on the eyeballs.

Rheumy Eyes

Wheat, rice, millets, as a matter of fact, all the cereals add to the amount of phlegm or mucus in the body. It is only vegetables, particularly greens, and fruit which can clear this condition. Eat more of them and less of cereals. Exercise is also essential. Wash the eyes frequently with cold water.

Trachoma

Poisonous humours in the body lead to trachoma and only a cleansing of the humours can help. Unless that is done, external applications, lotions and drugs will not be of much help.

Fruits, and vegetables clean the blood and refined foods like flour products, sugar, ghee, cereals, tea, coffee, cigarettes, condiments, produce morbid humours which give rise to disease. For two weeks eat only fruits and raw vegetables like tomatoes, carrot and spinach. Give up salt during above mentioned period. After that take to bread. boiled vegetables and fruits. Take an enema during the period when you live on fruits.

Conjunctivitis

Conjunctivitis or similar disorders which inflame the eyes and make them blood red are common among children.

The children should not be allowed to eat too much sweets. Their food should be simple and should include seasonal fruits and vegetables. If conjunctivitis or similar diseases strike, put them on a natural diet of fruits and vegetables; if they can take a salt-free diet it would further help get rid of this complication.

The eyes of sufferer should be washed thoroughly with lukewarm water using a cotton swab. A mud pack may be applied for half an hour twice daily. Cover the eyes with a thin cotton cloth and spread mud lightly over that. Keep the pack for ten to fifteen minutes. This will help ease the trouble. The clay used for mud pack should be absolutely clean.

Discoloured Eyes

Liver disorders, smoking and anaemia can lead to the whites of the eyes turning dirty. Give up smoking.

Night Blindness

This is a deficiency disease; if the elements needed are found in the diet night blindness will go. Natural salts and vitamins needed to make up the deficiency which causes night blindness are found in wholemeal bread, unmilled rice, fresh vegetables and unboiled milk. Put the child on a diet of these foods and ask him to eat at least 250 grammes of carrots each day. Carrot is a vegetable which contains vitamins which deal with the deficiency.

Dark Circles

The dark circles under the eyes may be due to malfunctioning of the liver and constipation. Late nights may also be a contributing factor. Reduce the amount of fats in the food; deal with your constipation first. Take plenty of exercise and spend restful nights. The dark circles will disappear soon.

Diseases of Teeth

The common problems of teeth are toothache, caries of the teeth, inflammation of the gums and pyorrhoea. All of them are produced from common causes like improper brushing, not chewing your food properly, dyspepsia, too much of intake of refined sugar and general neglect. Of these pyorrhoea is the most common and also the most serious. The regimen indicated for pyorrhoea will relieve other disorders also.

Pyorrhoea

This disease is characterised by the promotion of pockets of purulent material round the teeth and loosening of the affected teeth. It is a legacy of the modern civilisation with too much of emphasis on refined and canned foods, sugar, refined wheat flour and polished rice. In other words, it is the result of too little roughage in the diet and inadequate care of the teeth. Food tends to stagnate between the teeth leading to the excessive formation of tartar. There is a foul taste and also a foul odour in the mouth. A characteristic feature in the later stages is the tendency for the gums to bleed very often.

The sufferer should eat alkali-genic foods which are to be found in wheat flour not passed through a sieve, unpolished rice, unboiled milk, fresh fruit and raw, green vegetables. Lack of calcium leads to decay of teeth and give rise to the various diseases. Refined sugar, which does not contain any calcium needs it to be properly digested and takes the calcium from the bones to get assimilated into the system. The worst effect is, therefore, on the teeth. An adult needs ten grains of calcium in his daily diet which is available in flour, unpolished rice, banana, groundnut, coconut, green peas, almonds, figs, dates, cabbages, tomatoes, gourds, carrots, cucumber and spinach. It is also found in milk, sesame and oranges.

Exercises

Teeth also need exercise like other parts of our bodies. Hard foods like rusks, raw vegetables and hard-crusted fruits should be chewed in adequate quantities. Wheat soaked in water or maize roasted in sand could be taken in medium quantities to exercise the teeth. Germinated wheat would be still better because it contains Vitamin E, the specific for sterility among women, inadequate lactation among feeding mothers and miscarriages and slowly healing wounds.

Foods having Vitamin C, like lime and oranges, tomatoes, cabbage, onions, garlic, pineapple, grapes and the lowly myrobalan *(aanvala)* and guava should be particularly taken by those suffering from swollen or bleeding gums. Rubbing of the gums with the finger tips is also beneficial.

Steam Treatment

In case of swollen or bleeding gums if nothing else helps then steam treatment is quite helpful. Keep a vessel filled with water on heat and cover it with a lid with a small opening. When the steam starts escaping, expose your gums to its action. Intersperse the steam with rinsing your mouth with cold water. If the steam affects the face also, all the better. Apply fresh lime juice mixed with coconut or mustard oil after steaming it at night.

Brushing

Brush the teeth with a twig of the *neem* or acacia tree. Brush your teeth in the morning and, the last thing before you go to sleep. Remember that most of the mischief is done by the food particles which infest the crevices between the teeth which give rise to putrefaction. Do not use any tooth picks or other sharp sticks to pick your teeth. Munch a piece of radish, carrot, cucumber, apple or gauva after meals. That would be quite helpful in cleaning your teeth.

Blisters in the Throat

This complication points out accumulation of morbid humours in the system. Cleanse the system and take to a natural diet of fruits and vegetables. Start with fasting for one or two days followed by a diet of fruits in the morning and another type in the evening; for example, take oranges in the morning and papaya and guava for lunch. Eat tomatoes for dinner. One must drink about two litres of water during this period. Take a lukewarm enema daily. After the initial period of a diet of fruits, start taking whole meal bread and boiled vegetables.

You lose some weight in the initial period but that will not affect your capacity for work. Take more vegetables and fruits after you have completed the course of treatment.

Salivation During Sleep

This is an indication of bad digestion. Live on fruits alone for three to four days. Take an enema daily for about a week. Eat sparingly and take exercise. Excessive salvation will stop gradually.

Salivation (Excessive)

Some people suffer from excessive salivation. Sometimes, they have to swallow the saliva and interrupt their conversations to do it, otherwise thev spray saliva on the listeners.

Excessive salivation is due to too much of refined food and defective digestion of those substances. Reduce the amount of refined flour products, milled rice and sugar. Take exercise regularly, take long walks. The salivation will become normal after some period.

Nosebleed

Those children whose diet is lacking calcium, suffer from nosebleed. If the diet includes milk, oranges, green vegetables and other calcium bearing substances nosebleed will automatically vanish after some period.

After nosebleed wash the face of the child with cold water. A bandage half an inch thick and two inches broad should be wetted with water and applied to the spinal column of the sufferer from nosebleed for fifteen to twenty minutes to give immediate relief.

Snoring

Persons who generally sleep in a supine position throughout are liable to snore. Try sleeping on your side. That will reduce the severity of snoring.

Ringing in the Ears

Ringing in the ears may be caused by many factors like chronic catarrh, raised blood pressure or too much of quinine. You can get relief after you have taken treatment for these maladies and stop the use of quinine at once.

Pus from the Ear

Avoid foods which raise the amount of phlegm in the body, e.g. milled rice, sugar and lentils. You should take wholemeal bread, vegetables and fruits. Should take part in sports and games and should take regular exercise. Fresh air is of vital importance as is sun bathing. Sit in the sun so that sunlight penetrates the inner part of the ear for fifteen minutes. This process will help in stopping the discharge of pus from ear.

Numbness (In Hands and Feet)

Some people suffer from numbness of hands and feet. If they sit cross-legged for some time or hold something with the hands, it can produce numbness in the feet and hands. On changing position, there is a feeling of tingling which goes after some time.

These symptoms indicate defective circulation of blood. Have somebody massage patient's body for some days. He should take exercise regularly and take one to two litres of water in 24 hours. Rub body with hot water as he takes a hot bath. Immediately thereafter he should take a cold bath. The duration of the hot bath should be ten minutes and that of a cold bath only two minutes.

Morning Lethargy

This complication is a typical case of dyspepsia. One should take to a diet of boiled vegetables and fruits, and should also flush stomach twice in a week, by taking about a litre of lukewarm water with about 50 grammes of salt after visiting the toilet. One should vomit out all the water immediately after ingestion. If one takes to fruits only for a few days and takes an enema so long he is on fruits, it will be extremely beneficial.

Headache

This complication is usually the result of a malfunctioning intestine. See to it that you do not suffer from constipation; if you do, treat that condition first. Never take a pain killer for a headache, as that is likely to be more harmful in the future.

There is permanent cure for headaches in hydropathy. Start it with a diet of fruits for three to four days cleansing your bowels with a daily enema. On the fourth day take wholemeal bread and boiled vegetables for dinner. Take a hip bath in the morning and evening. The period of the hip bath should be increased gradually bath in the morning instead of a hip bath. The bathing of the genitals should be for ten minutes and gradually increase the time up to fifteen minutes. Start taking cow's milk in the evening with dinner when you undertake genitals bath. Initially take it for ten minutes but gradually increase the period to fifteen minutes. Supplement your diet with cow's milk when you take to genitals bath. This bath should be continued for a month. During this period of six to eight weeks the headache will leave you permanently.

During the period of above regimen, whenever you feel constipated take an enema. Take sun bath once a week: sit in the sun till you perspire freely. If it is too hot, cover your head with a wet towel. A cold bath immediately after a sun bath is also recommended.

Backache

This may trouble you due to many reasons. Disorders which cause it should be tackled first. Gout, constipation, a wrong posture and menstrual disorders of women can cause backache. If the pain persists even after these maladies have been cured, hot fomentation and massaging the affected part can help because in that case the ache may be due to the accumulation and massage will dispel the blood and give relief.

Weakness after Urination

After passing urine some people feel lethargic and weak. These symptoms indicate diabetes which is a disease of assimilation. Strengthening the digestion can cure it.

Heat Stroke

Do not forget to drink plenty of water before you venture outside in the sun during summer. Heat stroke is generally preceded by dehydration. Never try to suppress your thirst. Adequate intake of water and other liquids is essential in summer.

If head is covered with a wet towel when you have to go out in the sun, heat will never bother. Wear a hat or cap. It is better to cover your head from the rays of the sun during the noon-day sun which is rather severe in summer.

Heart Diseases

The main function of the heart is to pump the blood into the arteries and send the blood returning from the various organs with carbon dioxide to the lungs for purification purpose.

Heart is subjected to quite a few complications. The heart it never stops till death. The main causes of heart disease are the diseases of the coronary arteries (which nourish the heart muscle), high blood pressure and syphilis. Acute rheumatism—a predominantly infantile disorder—is responsible for most cases of heart disease occurring between the ages of 5 and 45 years. Other causes of heart disease are disorders like diphtheria, diseases of the thyroid gland and certain forms of chronic lung ailments. A small, but important group of heart diseases is due to the congenital abnormalities of the heart. In those disorders for example, the malformation of the valves or cavities in the valve developed in the mother's womb, the only recourse is to heart surgery. Certain deficiency diseases like beri-beri.

The heart to adjust according to the changes in the mode of living of its owner, known as compensation, is one of the vital factors which prolong life in spite of maladies to which this main organ is susceptible. This adjustment sometimes enables a person to go through life without suspecting the disease which invade the heart. It is a common fallacy to suppose that heart disease ends in sudden death. A man with a defective heart may live long, if he takes precautions. It is only when the heart muscle has become weakened due to some other illness, for example, diabetes, that the end may come suddenly. Another cause of sudden death by heart failure can be ascribed to the formation of a clot in the blood (thrombosis). Hardening of the arteries may lead to failure of the heart.

Major Ailments

The vast categories of heart ailments are: (i) those caused by inflammation of the muscle, the outer covering or the inner covering of the heart; (ii) hardening of the arteries and formation of a clot which may result in sudden interruption of the functioning of the heart; (iii) weakening of the muscle or degeneration of the organ because of advancing years: (iv) involvement of the heart as a corollary to rheumatism or syphilis; and (v) functional disorders like techycardia, bradicardia (an abnormally quick or slow pulse), blood pressure or hypertension and arrhythmia (lack of rhythm in the heart beat) and angina pectoris (pain in the chest, behind the sternum) and a sense of approaching death.

With the help of naturopathy the heart diseases can be cured safely and in a better manner. The only exception, it may be stated here, is congenital defects of the heart for which surgical interference is necessary after the "compensation" fails to relieve the condition.

The same course of treatment which is given in angina pectoris would help other heart ailments too regardless of the technical name given to them.

Angina

This complication is characterised by a sharp pain in the chest (behind the sternum) which leaves the victim breathless. There is a sense of impending doom. It is generally caused by the constriction of the main artery that leads into the heart, because of its hardening or deposition of fat in the insides. The pain radiates to the back, the shoulders and the arms, particularly the left arm. The attack may come on after a hearty meal, a sudden over-exertion or excitement or intense grief.

The true pain of angina has a tendency to spread to the shoulders and the arms. There is a constriction in the chest and profuse sweating. True angina must be differentiated from false or pseudo-angina which is of a nervous origin.

Medicine taken to relieve angina only help to make the condition more chronic. Patients taking recourse to traditional methods of treatment would be seen carrying tablets of nitro-glycerine to relieve the pain. The drug may be taken in an emergency but the correct treatment for angina begins when it is aimed at building the general health level of the sufferer.

When an attack is underway, the best thing is to apply hot towels over the heart region. That will relieve the constriction around the chest by dilating (through heat) the clogged artery which finds it difficult to pass the required amount of blood through it to the heart.

Treatment

The first step to deal with heart disease is to start a cleansing diet because the cleaner the blood, the less will be the chance of any toxicity building up around the region of the heart. The patient should subsist on a diet of fruit and fresh vegetables. His breakfast should consist of two oranges, an apple and grapes. For lunch he should take salad of lettuce, grated carrots and beetroot together with some boiled vegetables and bread made out of wholemeal flour. Fats, particularly saturated ones like ghee, should be banned and only a pat of butter—preferably fresh and not the tinned variety is recommended.

Salt should be avoided totally or taken in small quantities if the patient cannot avoid it.

If the sufferer prefers a non-vegetarian diet, he should eat steamed fish or boiled white meat. Fatty portions of meat, particularly pork, should be avoided. He should never overload his stomach because distension of the organ by flatulence or overloading may depress the diaphragm and the pain of angina may appear.

The patient of heart disease should fast for a short period according to their bodily strength so that the system is not overtaxed. Ailments like indigestion should not be allowed to arise as they are likely to tax the heart. A heart patient should eat so sparingly that he should feel hungry all the time. The last meal of the day should be taken at least three hours before going to bed in the night.

Enema should be taken recourse to in case of constipation. A short walk in the morning and evening is beneficial. Even traditional doctors have come to realise now that walking is the best exercise for a heart patient. Some of them even recommend jogging. A medical fact which should be stated here is that when you are walking, the pressure on the heart is reduced to some extent because the blood going back for purification through the heart to the lungs flows back more easily when you are walking than when you are sitting or lying down. Epsom salt bath should be taken once or twice in a week.

A patient must have a strict regimen of living in addition to eating. He must avoid stress, worry and excessive physical strain. If he has been on drugs before turning to naturopathy, they should be gradually withdrawn. A sudden stoppage of drugs is not recommended.

The above mentioned regimen should be followed in all cases of heart disease regardless of their technical name given by the experts

High Blood Pressure

This complication is called hypertension also, is the most common form of high blood pressure. Its causes include kidney disease, disorders of the endocrine glands and malfunctioning or disorders of the arteries. A congenital abnormality of the aorta is one of the most serious forms of hypertension. Its chief symptoms are headache, usually in the back of the head, ringing in the ears, giddiness. Headache is worst at the time of waking in the morning and it has a tendency to vanish during the day.

The hypertension runs its natural course, it usually causes death in the end as a result of heart failure. A proportion of the victims die of kidney failure and some of a stroke. The earlier the onset of hypertension, the poorer is the life expectancy. A large number of deaths supposed to have occurred from heart disease were really the handiwork of hypertension left unattended.

Hypertension can be either functional or organic: the latter is the case when the fatty substances accumulate in the smaller arteries carrying blood to the heart. The openings being smaller, the heart has to beat faster and exercise more pressure to supply the blood to the various organs. Hence the higher blood pressure.

Hypertension is a disease of the modern times. The fast life, the mental and physical pressures under which man in the present industrial and metropolitan environment works, gives rise to psychological tensions. Worry is known to increase the adrenalin in the blood stream which causes the pressure of the blood to go up. Hypertension makes its victim a less than useful member of society. He cannot do any serious work, feels tired and out of sorts all the time. Never does he have a feeling of freshness even if he has full sleep. Difficulty in breathing may be experienced by him and dyspepsia troubles him very often.

Very little physical work, a sedentary life, too much of intoxicants, tea, coffee, refined foods, destroy the natural pace of life. The expulsion of waste and poisonous matter from the body is hampered and the arteries and the veins become slack.

A healthy person should have a systolic pressure (at the best of the heart) of 100 mm plus age and the diastolic pressure (between the beats of the heart) should be 80 mm plus age. The blood pressure is accurately measured by an instrument known as *sphygmomanometer*. The pressure, if it is abnormally high, is accompanied by disease of the arteries. The blood pressure normally increases with the advance of age, due to the hardening of the arteries. But it is an indication of ill health; if one is healthy, the normal systolic blood pressure should range between 120 to 140 mm of Hg. and diastolic should range between 70 to 80 mm of Hg. whatsoever the age is after 20 years.

Kidney problems, hardening of the arteries and severe constipation leading to absorption of morbid humours through the gut lead to high blood pressure. Smoking is another addiction which leads to hypertension. Smoke a cigarette and then have your blood pressure taken: it will be some points more than the normal.

Treatment

The medicine prescribed by traditional physicians may temporarily reduce blood pressure, but they are harmful in the final analysis. The best way to reduce it is to remove the real cause. High pressure of blood is only a symptom of the poisonous matter which causes it and the naturopathic way of dealing with it is to remove the poisons from the system. Again, the ingestion of fresh fruits and vegetables instead of a traditional diet is helpful in ridding the body of the poisons which cause high blood pressure. A hypertension patient, if he is not too weak, should start the process of healing by living on fruits and vegetables for at least a week. The best course would be to take only fruits at five hourly intervals only thrice in the day. Breakfast should consist of oranges, lunch of guava and dinner of tomatoes, or apples. Fruits like oranges, apples. pears, mangoes, guava, pineapples, rose apples, raspberry. musk melon are the best diet in such cases. Bananas and jackfruit should be avoided. After a week of "fruits only" diet, milk should be added. Milk should preferably be of cow or goat and should be fresh. It should be boiled only once. After two weeks, the patient can be permitted cereals in his food. The porridge would be best.

Vegetables are also beneficial for a patient of high blood pressure, A salt-free diet is the best; but if you must take it, take it 25 per cent of the normal quantity. Vegetables should preferably be raw. If they are cooked, cook them with the rind on and do not let their natural juices burn in the process of cooking vegetables like cucumber, carrot. tomatoes, onion, radishes, cabbage and spinach are best taken in their raw form. They may be cut into small pieces and sprinkled with a little bit of salt and the juice of a lemon added to them in order to make more tasty.

The next step is to deal with a constipated bowel. During the period that fruits are the mainstay of the patient, he should take a warm water enema every day in order to clear his bowels.

If the patient is unable to take exercise, let him massage his body: otherwise he should take exercise. Massage should be away from the heart and towards the limbs and their extremities.

When the blood pressure shows signs of abating, take more exercise. Avoid too much straining of the heart, Breathe deeply while you are walking or doing exercise.

Rub your body with a rough towel vigorously for five to seven minutes after you have taken your bath. Avoid too cold water; add a little warm water to bring it to body temperature. If you have the patience, rub your body. instead of using a towel use your palms for extra benefit.

Early to bed is another cardinal principal which a person suffering from hypertension must follow. He should get eight hours of restful sleep. Those who find it difficult to sleep can keep their feet in warm water for 10 to 15 minutes and then wash them with cold water.

The high blood pressure patient must avoid over-straining, worries, tension, anger and haste. He must try to be cheerful. The natural treatment may take some time, but do not lose patience because it is the safest and the best way to get rid of this complication.

Palpitation

Some persons suffer from palpitation but doctors assure them that there is nothing wrong with their heart, but their medicines also do not help. What should be done in such condition?

Indigestion, constipation and flatulence can raise the pulse rate. Persons facing this complication should eat sparingly, take more organic foods so that is no danger of constipation or indigestion.

The sufferer should take deep breaths. Lie down on the bed, let all tensions and worries drain out of his system and relax his body completely. His pulse rate will automatically come down. If he is a smoker he must give up smoking, or if that is not possible, reduce smoking. He should avoid his intoxicating liquors also.

Anaemia

This is a condition where the amount of blood in the body is less than normal. Its main symptom is paleness of skin, a wan face, disinclination towards work of any kind, loss of appetite, etc. In order to understand its ramifications, a look at the composition of the blood is essential. The blood consists, in addition to the fluid, of corpuscles, minute bodies of the size of eight thousandth part of an inch. They are red corpuscles, white corpuscles and platelets. In the blood are also the various salts and proteins which nourish the tissues and also the waste products like uric acid which must be removed from the body. The red corpuscles act as carriers of oxygen. Every cubic millimetre of blood contains five million red blood corpuscles. The white corpuscles are the minute warriors which nature has equipped the blood with. Their main function is to fight infection.

There are many factors which cause anaemia, the main among them are: loss of blood due to injury, menstruation in excessive quantities, haemorrhage from piles: defective blood production due to infections, toxins, and drugs, inadequate intake and absorption of iron.

Treatment

Allopaths administer iron and Vitamin B_{12} in this condition the vital need of strengthening the constitution so that it can manufacture these elements for the body's needs. The complication affects mostly the young people. It is caused by wrong kind of living, irregular hours, addiction to smoking and drinking and almost no exercise. With anaemia come diseases like constipation, dyspepsia and nervous disorders. Palpitation and flatulence may also follow the onset of anaemia. Men may suffer from night emissions and the women from scanty discharge during menstruation period.

Iron, available in vegetable greens, bran of wheat, raisings, carrot, dates and oranges. The ingestion of these foods is a essential to deal with this complication.

The patient should start light exercise to tone up the system. Sun bathing in the morning for about a quarter of an hour daily is also a way to store up the elements that fight anaemia.

Massages are also quite helpful in anaemia. The patient must bathe in cold water in the morning and rub his body dry with the palms of his hands.

Person suffering from amaemia must have his full quota of sleep and remain cheerful. Anaemia born out of diseases like chronic malaria, bleeding piles, syphilis or loss of blood due to injury can be cured only if those diseases are treated first.

Jaundice

The yellow discolouration of the skin in jaundice occurs due to the deposition of the bile pigment in its deeper layers. It is usually the result of malfunctioning of the liver.

The liver is like a big chemical factory. The heat produced by the chemical changes taking place in it form an important contribution to the warming of the body. It secretes bile, the chief constituents of which are the bile salts, the pigment, cholesterol and lecithin. Besides producing bile, it forms red blood corpuscles, manufactures the fibrinogen of the blood and stores iron and corpuscles. The liver detoxicates noxious products made in the intestine and absorbed in the blood. It stores carbohydrate in the form of glycogen. It forms Vitamin A and is a storehouse of Vitamin B, and in the storage and metabolism of fat, it plays an extremely important role. Obstruction of the bile ducts which discharge bile salts and pigment into the intestine cause jaundice. The bile then gets mixed with the blood and gives a yellow pigmentation to the skin of the whole body. The obstruction could be due to gall stones or inflammation of the liver (hepatitis) caused by some infection or chronic malaria or ameobiosis. The seriousness of jaundice would depend, in the ultimate analysis, on the severity of the disease which has caused it in the first place. Pernicious anaemia and snake poisoning can also cause jaundice. Certain infective diseases like yellow fever, malaria, typhoid fever and pyaemia can also cause jaundice. The jaundice caused by acute yellow atrophy of the liver is the most serious form of the disease and is generally a killer.

The yellow colour of jaundice can be seen first in the white of the eyes and later over the whole skin. The urine is of a dark greenish-brown colour and the tongue is furred with a foul taste in the mouth. The stools are of grey or white colour and constipation is present in a severe form. Slowness of pulse and mental confusion may be present in long-continued cases. The patient may feel irritation all the time. There is also loss of appetite and apathy to food.

The attack of jaundice may begin by loss of sleep, appetite, irritation and dyspepsia. There may also be pain, a little below the right shoulder. The patient may feel chilly all over and have a feeling of nausea too. This is because of the fact that the liver loses the capacity to dissolve the fat into nutriment.

Fondness of foods made from fried foods, refined wheat flour, condiments, savouries which are highly spiced. produce the condition which ultimately leads to jaundice. because they constipate the bowel and the patient takes to purgatives. Some of the purgatives contain extract of mercury which further damages the functioning of the liver.

Treatment

To deal efficiently with jaundice see to it that the burden on the liver is reduced. The best course will be fasting and that will not mean starving the patient. If ingestion of food is stopped, the excretion of waste and morbid matter can be encouraged by freeing the system of the burden of digestion process.

Fasting for long periods is best done under the supervision of an experienced naturopath. Warm water enema after the improvement in the condition becomes apparent—that would be evident from the healthy pink. colour of the tongue—fresh fruit juice can be consumed. After a couple of days fresh fruit can be eaten instead of regular meals. Fruits, vegetables and foods which help the bowel to move properly should form the most essential part of the diet of a person who wants prevention against jaundice. Fats should be totally banned so long as the attack of jaundice lasts. After the virulence has abated. whole meal flour, boiled vegetables and salads can be allowed. Juice of a lime may be mixed with lukewarm water and taken in the morning and raisins, figs and fresh ripe fruits should become mainstay of the breakfast.

Stretching exercises are particularly useful for the jaundice patients. The best exercise would be walking on all fours—with both hands and feet. It activates the liver and increases the flow of bile. It also helps in digestion process.

Mumps

This problem is common among children. There is inflammation in the throat and severe pain. The patient also suffers from high temperature.

The children whose intake of water is insufficient and who suffer from constipation fall prey to this complication. Children should be encouraged to take adequate amounts of water and should visit the toilet regularly so that they do not develop constipation. Their diet should include sufficient amounts of fruits and vegetables. After the disease strikes them, they should be given an enema daily and should be kept on a diet of fruit juices. The inflamed part of the throat should be covered with a hot compress for ten minutes followed by a cold compress to be applied for one to two hours. Three to four days regimen mentioned above will deal with the problem.

Boils

Sometimes small boils appear on body which are extremely painful. In some cases the boils appear on hands and feet and scratching results in their bursting.

Wherever the boils are, but their cause is the same. They are due to the morbid humours in the body which are not being properly expelled. All of you must take to a diet of fruit for some days. Eat one kind of fruit thrice daily according to how hungry you feel. Take enema also during the days you are on a diet of fruit. Continue it for three days and on the fourth day adopt the following regimen: take half a litre of hot water with about 50 millilitres of juice of lime in the morning after stools. Take soup of vegetables for breakfast, boiled vegetables for lunch and fruits for dinner. Take raisins or figs (about 100 grammes) also with your dinner. Continue it for a week and then start taking bread with boiled vegetables. If you can keep it for a few weeks, boils will disappear automatically.

Gout

This is a disease of the joints and is a form of rheumatism. It is a constitutional disorder connected with excess of uric acid in the blood manifesting itself by inflammation of joints with deposition of urate of soda and also by morbid changes in various main organs. Gout occurs most commonly in spring and autumn, and this is a fact that women are less liable to it than men. Uric acid is formed in the system in the process of nutrition and is excreted by the kidneys. In a patient suffering from gout, the quantity of uric acid is found to be much more than normal. In a paroxysm of gout, the body appears to get rid of a lot of uric acid and there appears to be some relief but that is purely temporary.

Gout is believed to be hereditary since it has been found in 50 to 80 per cent of the cases that the patient's parents or grand-parents suffered from the diseases. The disease affects the persons who avoid exercise of any kind more than those who lead active lives, but it is not always true. On the other hand, inadequate exercise, fondness of rich foods and especially alcohol are the precipitating factors in the onset of the disease. Though some teetotallers and vegetarians are also found to fall prey to gout.

The onset of this problem is more common in mature age. Persons exposed to the influence of lead poisoning such as plumbers are apt to suffer from gout. Attacks of the disease are readily excited by disorders of digestion. fatigue, injuries to particular joints, and exposure to cold.

This disease strikes without warning or there may be premonitory symptoms. Among the most common of these are disorders of the digestive organs, with a feeble and capricious appetite, flatulence, uneasiness in the right side in the region of the liver, and irritation in the urinary organs. There is also irritability numbness and coldness in the limbs. The attack comes usually at night. usually between two and three in the morning. The affected part is found to be swollen and of a deep red colour. The skin is tense and glistening and the surrounding veins are more or less distended. The attack lasts for a week or ten days during which the patient suffers from constipation. dyspepsia and extreme thirst. The urine is scantly and high coloured with a copious deposit. consisting chiefly of urates. The joint affected may become swollen but if the disease is not attended to, the swelling spreads to other joints and it becomes chronic. Joints also become enlarged and refuse to function without causing severe pain.

Just like all other diseases, gout is the result of inadequate excretion of the morbid and poisonous matter from the orifices of the body. If they become slack and do not function properly, those substances accumulate in the body and produce gout. Life depends on healthy blood and nature has devised catarrh, diarrhoea and fevers to force the human system to expel the accumulated waste matter. If these diseases are suppressed, as happens in most cases when the patient takes to allopathic treatment, the poisonous and morbid matter attacks the part of the body which is weaker than others. And that is the main cause of chronic diseases.

The main cause is the type of food which we are addicted to. Our blood is chiefly alkaline and anything that tends to produce acidity should be avoided. In other kinds of treatments, the real cause of the diseases if not attacked and recourse is taken to pain killers or antidoting of the poison is undertaken. The Ayurvedic practitioners prohibit the intake of fruits and vegetables on the plea that they may produce cold which is supposed to be bad for the gout and thus deprive the patient of the real cure. Some physicians advise patients to have their teeth or tonsils extracted under the misconception that the seat of the disease lies there. But even the excision of these never give any type of relief.

Treatment

First of all, ensure that all the orifices of the body which expel waste and morbid matter are activated to do their work properly. The patient should breathe fresh air, so that oxygen is available to him in larger quantities to cleanse his blood of poisonous humours. The patient must increase his intake of water to produce more urine. He should take lukewarm water in the morning and evening mixed with the juice of lime. The pores of the skin should be activated by a cold bath every day and drying of the body with vigorous rubbing with the palms of the hand. If the pain in the joints is too severe and the patient is unable to massage his body himself, he should seek help of somebody else. The patient should take sunbath also. The head may be covered with a wet towel to save it from excessive heat of the sun. Half an hour in the sun will activate the sweat glands. A cold bath is beneficial after a sun-bath or he should wipe his body with a wet towel. Sun-bathing should be done no more than thrice in a week. If there is no sun, sweat should be induced by a steam bath or by merely soaking one's feet in hot water by applying proper method.

Patient's food should consist of fresh fruits and vegetables. Fruits can be taken without peeling should be taken. In the beginning of the treatment, the best course would be to live on fruit juices. That would give some rest to the intestines. Fruits recommended are: grape fruit, oranges, pineapple, raspberry and pear. Vegetables like the various gourds, cabbage, tomatoes and greens are the best. The more chronic the disease, the greater should be the period for which the patient should live on vegetables and fruits.

After a five days regimen during which only fruits and vegetables are taken, milk should be added to the diet. It should preferably be boiled and taken in quantities of 250 to 500 millilitres at one time. Bread should be taken only after a fortnight of living on fruits and vegetables. Potatoes can be taken in place of bread with advantage as they contain more alkaline matter.

Hot fomentation recommended to reduce the pain in the joints. About 75 grammes of salt should be added to one litre of hot water for fomentation. The site of fomentation should be washed with cold water later on. Those who suffer from a constant pain should apply a paste of raw potatoes ground find on the affected joints the paste should be allowed to remain for some hours on painful area.

Goitre

Bronchocele or goitre is a term applied to the swelling on the front of the neck caused by the enlargement of the thyroid gland. It is caused by deficiency of iodine in the diet. It is an endemic disease prevalent in the hill areas of the country. The growth of the thyroid gland is generally unattended by pain but if the goitre becomes large it may cause hoarseness. Too enlarged a goitre may interfere with breathing and the swallowing.

Goitre can be dealt efficiently by taking foods which contain natural iodine. They are pineapple, water nut (*singhara*), lotus reed and stem of the lotus.

Filaria and Hydroseal

Both of the diseases are endemic in Gaya and Patna. Arms and legs swell to elephantine proportions in filaria.

These two diseases are caused by milled rice. Most of the people in the area have a diet which consists mainly of this rice which is devoid of natural salts and vitamins. A diet of fruit and vegetables with minimum of cereals will be beneficial for the sufferer.

Elephantiasis

Some persons complain that their legs swells if they pedal a cycle, walk or even sit on a chair or on a bed with their legs hanging down. And no treatment gives them any relief.

Elephantiasis is caused by the accumulation of morbid humours in the body. It can be cured by a massive cleansing process of the whole body. Fasting will give relief in many cases. Prolonged fasting may be difficult for one, but if he can fast one day in the week, it would gradually give relief. One must consume two to three litres of water on the day of fasting. He must take an enema on the evening of the fast and on the morning after. Adopt a natural lifestyle. Take exercise regularly. The food should include wholemeal bread, green vegetables and fruits. If one can take a salt-free diet, it will be highly beneficial for him.

Obesity

Corpulence or obesity is a condition of the body characterised by over-accumulation of fat under the skin and around particular internal organs. While the state of health differs from person to person, other things being equal, the fatter a person is the slower he will be. Doctors and actuaries have calculated the weight that a person of a particular height should have and anybody having a weight much above the average is likely to be unhealthy and would have a lower life expectancy. It has been proved from experience that the fat persons have a greater chance of dying early than those of average weight. There are several cases where extremely overweight people did not live beyond their thirties and died prematurely.

The obesity may be due to the disturbances of some of the endocrine glands, like the thyroid, pituitary and the sex glands. In some families obesity is transmitted from one generation to the other, but in most cases it is the direct result of a life of ease and over-eating. A luxurious inactive or sedentary life is a well recognised predisposing cause. The more immediate cause is over-eating and excessive intake of liquor. The indulgence in food beyond what is required to repair the daily waste goes towards the increase of fat. Those addicted to liquor are particularly affected if they eat a normal diet since what is not generally realised is that alcohol meets the immediate energy needs of the body and the food that is eaten is deposited in the form of fat. Particularly guilty in this respect is the intake of fatty, sugary and starch foods. Alcoholic liquors, particularly beer, contain sugar and contribute to the deposition of fat on the body making life miserable for the sufferer.

Ladies are more prone to obesity, particularly after child-birth in our country, because the new mother is fed on fatty and starchy foods under the impression that the blood loss attendant on delivery must be made up by extra-rich diet.

Excessive obesity cannot be called healthy condition, because the increase in the bulk of the body, rendering exercise more difficult, leads to tension and defective nutrition of the muscle, while the accumulations of fat in the chest hinders the functions of the various organs of the body. The mental activity of the corpulent tends to be impaired, although there have been exceptions to this rule. It is an established fact that health cannot be maintained for long period under excessive obesity.

The fat persons fall victim much more readily to serious diseases like diabetes, gall-stone, arterial disease, high blood pressure and varicose veins. According to a survey report, an increase of 25 pounds above standard weight reduce the life expectancy of a man of 45 by 25 per cent.

There should be a weight-energy ratio, the more obese a person is, the more energy his body consumes merely to maintain itself and the sum of energy left for other activities is proportionately reduced. For example, those who live by manual labour seldom suffer from corpulence: it is the leisured class, with nothing much to do but too much to eat who become fat and troubled by disease.

Obesity is like constipation: just as waste accumulates in the gut, matter which should not have been accumnlated in the body tends to gather in the form of fat on the various organs. Skin is stretchable, hence, fat accumulates in layers upon layers under the skin.

Treatment

To avoid getting fat in the first place is better than reducing. One would not have become obese if he avoids over-eating and does exercise. The battle against obesity has therefore, to be fought with courage and fortitude. Weight could be reduced by fasting in a limited time but that is not advisable. Sudden and total fasting may help the poison accumulated in the body to attack it fiercely. Fasting has to be gradual and systematic. The best course is to make fruits and boiled vegetable the mainstay of your diet. A diet of fruits and vegetables will give you the vitamins and the mineral salts for the sustenance of life, but would tend to reduce the amount of fat that has already been accumulated. The other method of reducing the fat is vigorous exercise. Foods tending towards acidity like meat, fish, eggs, refined flour, lentils, fats, polished rice should be totally banned in the case of obesity. Wheatever the patient eats should be bland, because seasoning and condiments tend to make the food more palatable increasing the danger of overeating. The fruits recommended are pineapples, raspberry, tomatoes, apples, pears, oranges papaya, musk melon and melon, in that order. The vegetables should be greens of all type, cucumber, gourds. etc. Tuberous edibles should be avoided. Only carrot may be taken.

After two weeks of the diet prescribed above, the patient can have wholemeal bread, a pat of butter and milk. The first thing in the morning that the corpulent should take is a glass of water to which a lime has been added. Salads should be permitted provided that salad oil or eggs have not been added. The best reducing agent in the present author's experience has been the juice of cucumber, gourd (bottle gourd—*lauki*) and tomatoes to which a lime and a spoonful of honey has been added. In between meals, cucumber and tomatoes can be taken as snacks in any quantity.

When one would follow the above-mentioned regimen, the weight will start going down, but the patient should not lose heart if the progress is slow in the beginning. A speedy reduction of weight is possible by vigorous exercise coupled with inadequate diet, but that might prove harmful to the general health of the patient. The best exercise is skipping the rope, and other exercise which strains the muscles can also be helpful.

Hip bath for 15 to 20 minutes in the morning and evening along with the diet and the exercise recommended would speed up the process of losing fat. Mud packs can also help, as well as sun-bathing for long enough to produce a sweat. Steambaths for the purpose of reducing corpulence are not recommended since the benefit is not permanent and too much of exposure to steam is likely to harm the nerve ends under the skin.

The best time to start slimming in India and other tropical conditions is the summer when a large variety of stresses help in the reduction of fat in the body of obese person.

Insufficient Lactation

In some cases the mother of newborn baby is unable to breast—feed her child, because there is not enough milk to slake the thirst of the infant and the child has to be fed with a bottle.

In such cases, if the diet of the mother is normal with salts and vitamins there is no reason why she should suffer from insufficient lactation and be not able to feed her baby. She should take only milk and fruits in the morning and evening and her lunch should consist of boiled vegetables and wholemeal bread. She should take long walks in the morning and evening. Her water intake should be at least one and a half to two litres per day.

Fat on the Abdomen

In some cases there are layer upon layers of fat on abdomen of ladies, the skin is criss-crossed with furrows.

It is natural that skin over the abdomen gets stretched during pregnancy and lack of exercise after child-birth results in accumulation of fat all over the abdomen. Hip baths and long walks can deal with the condition. Fast walking for five to seven kilometres, hip baths and a diet of vegetables and fruit can help in getting rid of excessive fat.

Nervous Disorders

These disorders are more difficult to diagnose than diseases of the various organs of the body because the nervous system is hidden from the eye of the physician and it can be known only from the disturbances of the organs governed by the affected nerves whether and of what type the nervous disease is. Under this head come forgetfulness, hysteria, mental defectiveness, apoplexy, mental illness, neuresthenia and others. The most common nervous disorder with which the layman is familiar is nervous weakness, nervous exhaustion or nervous breakdown.

There are various causes of nervous diseases. Some people are born with a nervous disposition and it is that category which generally suffers from headaches, neuralgia, hysterical manifestations and bizarre forms of mental activity. The nervous system is exposed to the hectic modern life which tends to bring on many diseases like anxiety states, digestive disturbances and exhaustion. Shocks to both mind and body such as the loss of somebody very dear, money reverses, an unfortunate love affair and an accident may be the root causes of many chronic nervous complaints. Certain organic poisons like the one produced in body by diseases like syphilis give rise to serious nervous disorders. Chronic alcoholism may bring on severe mental derangement. The organic diseases may be apparent from an autopsy but the inorganic disorders manifest themselves in the shape of anxiety, nervous breakdowns and hysteria.

Weak nervous system can give cause diseases like dyspepsia or palpitation which cannot be helped by remedies directed towards those organs. It is but natural since it is the brain and the nervous system enclosed in it which controls the bodily functions. A sudden loosening of bladder in case of fright is an example.

The person suffering from nervous disorder generally experiences a sense of agitation, perplexity, confusion, worry, nameless fear, disappointment, loneliness, irritability, and insomnia. The physical symptoms are dyspepsia, headaches, constipation, vague aches and pains all over the body and feverishness. The patient is also inclined to be a hypochondriac. The moment he reads about or hears the symptoms of a disease he imagines that he suffers from it. His well-wishers should not talk about ailment in his presence and should keep him away from any medical literatures.

The main cause of a nervous breakdown is the greed and lust for undue success—which again is measured in the good things of life—motivates a man to overwork, both mentally and physically. Constant worry about things being done and to be done lead to tension and a man falls prey to his imagination. Overstraining leads to mistakes which erodes his self-confidence and after that the only way is the way downhill.

Treatment

The sufferer must live a normal, natural life. He should try to get more sleep. During the day also he should be advised to relax on a bed for some hours. The loosening of tension by relaxation will help his organs to do their work properly and he would be able to overcome his problems.

The sufferer should start exercising regularly. He should take walks and if possible take to jogging. His food should include bread made from wheat from which bran has not been sieved out, fruits and boiled vegetables. Since nervous debility shows a marked lack of Vitamin B, the deficiency should be made up by inclusion in his diet of foods which contain it in larger measure. Unpolished rice, milk, cucumber, mangoes, pears, pineapples, guava, tomatoes, raisins and leafy vegetables should be his mainstay. He should be asked to eat his food in a relaxed manner, chewing it properly before swallowing.

Massaging can be of great help in reactivating the nervous system. Hydropathic treatment is also recommended and that merely consists in bathing his spine with a garden or bathroom shower for a couple of minutes. The water should be cold. During summer cold showering of the spine could be done three times or more and in winter twice would be sufficient.

The sufferer will have to exercise his willpower to deal with the disease. He must be told that he is getting better. Psychological impressions must be created on his mind which will help him to understand that his disease is not incurable. Suggestion is the best thing in such circumstances. It has to be remembered that certain nervous diseases like hysteria are the results of autosuggestion and nothing else.

Exercises

Sit on your feet with your stomach touching your knees. Try to keep your spine straight and extend both your arms. Then thrust your left foot forward and stand up with a jerk. Resume your earlier position and repeat the exercise with your right foot.

Stand upright with your right leg planted about a foot from your left. Join your hands and extend the arms downward, upward and then backward. Move the arms with the hands joined in a circular motion and inhale and exhale deeply during the movement.

Lie on your back on the floor with your elbows touching your sides. Then try to raise the body with your elbows and heels and then resume the former position.

Stand like a boxer, indulge in shadow boxing for some time, shuffling your feet as a boxer does.

Stand in the normal position and then sit down with a jerk on your toes, with your palms touching the ground. Suddenly jerk your legs back just as you were about to do push-up. The exercise is akin to doing sit-ups and push-ups at the same time. The above mentioned regimen if followed for some weeks, will deal with nervous disorder efficiently.

Insomnia

Sound sleep gives relief from tension, rest to the brain and the body and a person wakes up fresh and rejuvenated after sleep. But in some people the feeling of freshness is missing: they feel tired when they wake up. Some cannot sleep and others fall asleep the moment they lie on bed.

Sleeplessness or insomnia is a condition that often causes annoyance, and by depriving the person of natural rest produces interference with the full activity during the day-time. When it becomes a habit, it may form a serious menace to health of a person.

This complication may arise due to a variety of causes. and they may act so effectively as to keep the person awake altogether, or they may serve, when present in a less degree, to produce one of the forms of dreaming and unrefreshing slumber. Insomnia generally strikes persons of a nervous temperament, those who are given to intellectual overwork. Manual overwork may also produce the condition by throwing the nervous system out of gear. Bodily fatigue, however, generally acts as a sleep-inducing agent. In temporary cases of sleeplessness the cause is usually to be sought in some external source of irritation. Too much cold, or heat and humidity, or the presence of mosquitoes may interfere with sleep in some cases. A slight, nagging pain, or dyspepsia—in which pain may not be present in any appreciable degree may also interfere with sleep. Such temporary insomnia is easy to deal with: the moment the external cause that interferes with sleep is removed, it is cured but it is the chronic insomnia which is hard to deal with.

In conditions of habitual sleeplessness, a voluntary limitation of the hours of sleep, combined with overstudy, worry or grief, is often instrumental in forming a habit which is exceedingly difficult to break. The brain remains active despite the efforts of the person to compose himself for sleep. A similar state of matters is often the effect of poisonous materials circulating in the blood, as in fevers, gout, intemperance and over-indulgence in tobacco. Another cause of insomnia is neuresthenia. Persons suffering from it usually fall asleep the moment they get into bed but after an hour or two they wake up and connot sleep the whole night.

In nutshell, worry, thoughts, of sex, over-indulgence in smoking or drinking, late dinners, preoccupation with business or work even after working hours, airless bedrooms, playing of games like chess or cards before retiring to bed are some of the main causes of insomnia. Excessive noise in the surroundings is also bad for sleep. A person not having a clear conscience may also suffer from this complication.

How to Sleep Well

* One should stop thinking about anything but sleep half an hour before he gets into bed.

* Dinner time should be fixed and so should be the time when he gets into bed.

* He should not consume heavily spiced food, meat or liquor. Excessive smoking also makes one insomniac.

* A clean, airy bedroom and clean bed are extremely essential. The clothes in which one sleeps must also be loose and should not constrict any part of the body.

* One should compose himself for sleep. Get rid of all the worries about what he has done during the day or propose to do the next day.

Tranquillizers to induce sleep should be avoided since they are habit-forming. There are a large number of cases, particularly in the west, who are addicted to sleeping pills and whose need for greater and greater number of the pills goes on increasing. Drug-induced sleep is never as restful as the one that comes naturally. Drugs are likely to create more complications than they can remove they make one addict.

Treatment

The chronic cases can be dealt with only by resort to a natural diet of fresh fruit and vegetables, a daily regimen of exercise and freedom from worry or tensions. Light exercise of the neck and back muscles shortly before going to sleep can help. A four-inch broad water-soaked bandage tied to the neck can also be of great help.

Having a bath before sleep and rubbing body dry with your palms can also help induce sleep. A cup of hot water or hot milk can also help immediately before going to bed.

Sleeplessness because of mental excitement can be dealt by soaking feet in warm water. The temperature of the water should not be more than 3 to 4 degrees higher than body temperature. A damp towel soaked in cold water may be wrapped round the head. For more serious cases of sleeplessness, soaking the whole body in a tubful of warm water of body temperature is the remedy. If you can sleep lying in the bathtub for half an hour, it would give you the freshness that two hours sleep on the bed cannot provide.

In many cases, insomnia is due to lack of physical exercise. Physical exercise is the specific remedy for such cases.

Stammering

This is a condition in which a person hesitates in the act of speaking, being unable for a time to pronounce certain syllables or repeating the same syllable over and over again.

This complication is not due to any defect in the brain or in the speech organs, and may be described as a functional disease, or a bad habit, or a sign of diffidence. It begins in childhood and is a practice which one child learns from another, just as any peculiarity of speech in one person is liable to be unconsciously mimicked by another. The actual cause of stammering is lack of co-ordination between the various parts concerned in speech. The organs of speech are the chest, corresponding to the bellows of a harmonium, the larynx, corresponding to the keys and the changes in the mouth effected by the tongue, palate, lips, etc. which correspond to the stops of the organ which modulate the notes. Just as all the three parts of the organ must work in co-ordination, so should the chest, the larynx and the production of sound by the lips, the palate and the tongue.

Stammering is due to a nervous state and must be psychologically treated. The first step is to see that the nervous system is in perfect shape and is in full control of bodily functions as it should be. For that, one has to get rid of the malfunctioning of the body.

Treatment

A sufferer should give up smoking, or if that is difficult, reduce the quantum. That would, in itself, tone up the nervous system. No alcoholic beverages should be taken by a stammerer. Anything that excites the nervous system should be avoided.

Exercise in the open air is essential. Go for long walks, do anything which will make you to spend a lot of time in the open air.

In most cases, stammering starts with fear: a child might have been frightened in its infancy when shouted at; that might have produced a shock which gave rise to stammering in later life. One should try to get at the root of the problem and if it is a fear which has haunted the patient, the whole thing should be explained to him. A little bit of psychological approach, in fact psycho-analysis, is needed in such cases. The will power of the patient should be strengthened: he should be encouraged to introspect and rid himself of the fears which might have haunted him through childhood. The patient should learn to relax and rid himself of all the tensions which have plagued him. The best way to relax is to lie on your back in a secluded corner of the park or any open space. Let all thoughts of work or worldly worries drain out of your mind. Imagine that you are free from all mental and physical problem.

Inhale deeply while all your muscles are relaxed. Do not strain yourself while doing it: release your breath slowly. Repeat this process of deep inhaling and slow exhaling seven times. If this is continued for some weeks, stammering would disappear.

One should establish complete co-ordination between his mental and physical faculties. The above exercise will help achieve this coordination. Palpitation would cease and tensions will drain out of his system.

This complication is also due to thought in a lesser measure, lack of co-ordination among the three organs of speech. Establish that co-ordination. If there is any involuntary tremor in your tongue or jaw in the process of pronunciation, let it pass before you articulate your words. The best way to tone up the muscles of the jaw is to put your index finger in the throat and move your lower jaw. Move it slowly in a downward motion: relax the tension of the jaw muscles. Continue this exercise till the mouth does not open without your larynx coming into action.

One should sit with a mirror and let the light be on his back. Reflect the sunlight through the mirror into his open mouth. Breathe deeply and open his mouth slowly. Reflect the mirror on his tongue. It should be sticking the lower part of the mouth, if you have been doing your exercises properly. Loosen your tongue: it should never be stiff. If it is, stammering will result. Articulate the Hindi words *Kya ho*. It is a good exercise to improve the functioning of the tongue.

After going through the regimen described above for a fortnight or even a month, stand before a mirror for fifteen to twenty minutes and read something aloud. Breathe deeply before you begin, but you do not have to retain the breath for any length of time. Breathe slowly as you read. Pronounce each word consciously in a clear manner. If in this process, your face looks ridiculous do not mind it.

One should pronounce the syllables clearly—it will need a lot of effort in the beginning. He may be stopping at Ts and Bs or Ms. One should make a conscious effort to enunciate them clearly.

The stammerer should try to sing, those given to stammering usually do not stutter while they sing. Stammerer should try pronouncing sentences in a singsong manner and later on, he can correct himself.

One should be regular in the exercises suggested above. It is the regularity and the perseverance which will pay dividends. Increase gradually the time of the exercises. Take a sympathetic friend into confidence and read out aloud to him: ask for his suggestions and go on improving your elocution: you would soon overcome this problem.

Epilepsy

Falling sickness or epilepsy is a term applied to a nervous disorder characterised by a fit of sudden loss of consciousness, attended with convulsions. Although in most cases an epileptic attack comes on suddenly, it is in some cases atttended by certain premonitory indications or warnings which appear some time before the actual seizure. There may be a change in the disposition, such as an unusual elevation or depression of spirits, or some alteration in outlook. There are also some peculiar sensations which immediately precede the attack which are known to medicine by the name of *aura epileptica*. They are apparent in about half the cases of epileptic fits and may be in the form of pain in a limb or in some internal organ, such as the stomach. There may be an experience of a strange smell or vision. In some cases preliminary trembling of the limbs is noticed. Sometimes the warning symptoms appear sufficiently in advance to allow the patient to lie down or reach a place of safety before the seizure actually starts.

Epileptic seizure is usually preceded by a loud scream or cry. It is not, as was sometimes thought, to be a cry of pain or terror but merely a convulsive action of the muscles of the larynx and the expulsion of air through the throat. If the patient is standing he immediately falls and often sustains serious injury. The muscles become tense, the head is turned to one side and breathing is arrested for the moment. The face turns pale and then livid, the pupils are dilated and the pulse rapid. This is the first stage of the fit and lasts only for half a minute; later there is spasm of the muscles and the whole body is thrown into violent agitation. The eyes roll wildly and the teeth are gnashed, sometimes injuring the tongue. The breathing is noisy and sometimes blood tinged with foam issuing from the mouth of the stricken person. In some cases even the bowels and the bladder may be voided. This stage of the attack lasts from a few seconds to several minutes, after which convulsions subside and consciousness returns. After that there is a state of drowsiness and stupor which may continue for several hours. The patient may waken up either quite recovered or fatigued and depressed and occasionally in a state of excitement which sometimes assumes the form of mania.

The exact cause of the disease has not come in the light as yet, and all that can be said about the direct cause of the malady is that in the healthy brain, nerve energy is capable under control of will, of being expended in a sudden and explosive manner but in the epileptics uncontrolled discharges of energy, devoid of any purposive action, take place from time to time in an unusual manner.

Treatment

The modern medical science has not been able to cure the disease: the only palliative it offers is sedation. That may quieten the patient and the seizure may not be very virulent, but sedation is no cure.

With the help of naturopathy, the disease can be thoroughly cured without any danger of any relapse. The present author believes that the real cause of the disease is the poisonous matter which the body is unable to expel and which reaches the vital centres of the brain which control muscular activity. It has also been noticed that the disease strikes only those whose constitution is unable to deal with the waste matter produced in the body after the ingestion of refined foods or fried and overdone edibles. Prolonged lack of vitamins and minerals can also lead to the onset of the complication.

The treatment of epilepsy should start with fasting from one to three days in a week and then a diet of fruit and boiled vegetables without salt. During fasting only water and lime juice should be taken. The diet must be continued for at least four weeks before reverting to normal food. And then, even that normal food should not contain any condiments or over-refined substances. The more natural the form of the food, the better it is for keeping one in good health.

After getting up in the morning, the patient should vigorously rub his body with a dry towel and take a hot bath in a tub. The temperature of the water should not be above the body temperature and the patient must soak himself in the tub for half an hour. The spine should be given a hot bath and then a cold one. The best way to do it is to put a towel soaked in hot water over the spine for two minutes and then another towel soaked in cold water. The process should be repeated five times. Five sets of towels should be kept. The patient must live in an airy room.

After a month of the regimen suggested above, the patient can return to his previous diet, but care should be taken to see that no edibles are taken which may tend to excite any of the organs of the body. His diet should include: 50 per cent fruit, 25 per cent boiled vegetables, 10 per cent dried fruits or their kernels and 15 per cent cereals. Exercise which strains the muscles must be undertaken simultaneously.

An epileptic patient must avoid excitement of all types. His sex life must be severely restricted. Smoking, drinking and even tea and coffee should be prohibited as they cause excitement.

The patient should always remain cheerful and should not get disheartened. The disease is not incurable. It can be dealt efficiently with the help of naturopathy.

Polio

Polio is another name for infantile paralysis to which only children are prone. It is an infectious disease involving the spinal cord and the brain.

Polio is believed to be of a bacterial origin which has an incubation period of 3 to 21 days. The onset may be sudden or gradual. The child may be apathetic for some days and may complain of vague aches and pains in the various parts of the body. After that the paralysis of the limbs may come on suddenly with a sharp rise in temperature. The fever goes up to 103° F or even higher. The child may go to bed in a state of fever and may suffer a paralytic attack during sleep. The extent of the paralysis would depend on the extent to which the spinal cord and the brain are associated.

Naturopaths say that the cause of the disease is the loss of tone and power of the nerve centres in the spinal cord dealing with the co-ordination and activity of the muscles of the arms and legs, brought on by systematic wrong feeding, the absence of organic mineral salts so essential for the proper growth of the body. In laboratory experiments, guinea pigs fed exclusively on white bread, polished rice and other refined foods devoid of mineral salts start showing symptoms of infantile paralysis after a few weeks. When the diet is changed to wholemeal bread or unpolished rice rapid recovery is recorded.

Treatment

As long as the temperature does not come down to normal, the procedure adopted in other fevers should be followed. The child should fast and only water and orange juice in medium quantities should be given. In addition, massage of the affected limbs—preferably the whole body is recommended. Any oil—especially olive oil—can be used as a vehicle for massage. After recovery the child should be encouraged to spend as much time in the open, fresh air as possible. Fresh fruits and vegetables, together with unrefined foods in their natural condition, should be the mainstay of his diet.

Cold Feet

Some people suffer from cold feet and that keeps them awake in the nights.

This happens due to defective circulation of blood in the lower extremities. One must take exercise regularly and take more of vegetables and fruit. Wash the feet with cold water before going to sleep: the blood will rush to them to warm up the skin and the sufferer will get rid of this problem.

Nightmares

Some persons suffer from nightmares. There is a feeling of choking and they wake up drenched in perspiration.

Nightmares and disturbed are usually the result of an overfull stomach. Eat sparingly at night. Have your dinner three hours before you go to bed. Stop taking milk if that is the last thing you take at night. A light dinner of boiled vegetables and fruits will help cure the condition. Take vigorous exercise so that you are tired by the time you fall on bed. Take a few deep breaths before falling asleep. Relax every muscle in your body and tell yourself that you are not going to have nightmares.

Index